Medical Procedures, Testing and Technology

nova
Medicine & Health
New York

Medical Procedures, Testing and Technology

Vascularization and Its Role in Medicine and Tissue Engineering
Emre Bulbul, MD and Murat Oguz Ozilhan, MD
(Editors)
2023. ISBN: 979-8-89113-041-8 (Hardcover)
2023. ISBN: 979-8-89113-118-7 (eBook)

Chronic Disease Follow-Ups for Adults in Primary Care
Duygu Üstünol, MD (Editor)
Bahar Ürün Unal, MD (Editor)
2022. ISBN: 979-8-88697-050-0 (Hardcover)
2022. ISBN: 979-8-88697-138-5 (eBook)

Various Methods and Novel Techniques: Rapid Molecular Detection of Human, Plant, Genetic, and Microbial Infectious Diseases, Pathogenic Bacteria, and Organisms
Mohamad Hesam Shahrajabian, PhD (Author), Wenli Sun, PhD (Author)
2022. ISBN: 978-1-68507-721-1 (Softcover)
2022. ISBN: 978-1-68507-808-9 (eBook)

ELISA: Advances in Research and Applications
Jose Ma. M. Angeles, PhD (Editor)
2022. ISBN: 978-1-68507-500-2 (Hardcover)
2022. ISBN: 978-1-68507-594-1 (eBook)

Principles and Practices of Non-Invasive Mechanical Ventilation Monitoring: From Intensive Care to Home Care
Antonio M. Esquinas, MD, PhD (Editor)
2021. ISBN: 978-1-53619-689-4 (Hardcover)
2021. ISBN: 978-1-53619-850-8 (eBook)

More information about this series can be found at
https://novapublishers.com/product-category/series/medical-procedures-testing-and-technology/

Emre Bulbul, MD
and Murat Oguz Ozilhan, MD
Editors

Vascularization and Its Role in Medicine and Tissue Engineering

nova
Medicine & Health
New York

DOI: https://doi.org/10.52305/RBES3580

NOTICE TO THE READER

Library of Congress Cataloging-in-Publication Data

Names: Bulbul, Emre, editor. | Oguz Ozilhan, Murat, editor.
Title: Vascularization and its role in medicine and tissue engineering / Emre Bulbul, MD (editor), Department of Urology, Vakfikebir State Hospital/Trabzon, Turkey, Murat Oguz Ozilhan, MD (editor), T.C. Ministry of Health Ankara City Hospital, Ankara, Turkey.
Description: New York : Nova Science Publishers, [2023] | Series: Medical procedures, testing and technology | Includes bibliographical references and index. |
Identifiers: LCCN 2023035508 (print) | LCCN 2023035509 (ebook) | ISBN 9798891130418 (hardcover) | ISBN 9798891131187 (adobe pdf)
Subjects: LCSH: Prevascularization. | Neovascularization.
Classification: LCC R857.P74 V37 2023 (print) | LCC R857.P74 (ebook) | DDC 612/.028--dc23/eng/20230808
LC record available at https://lccn.loc.gov/2023035508
LC ebook record available at https://lccn.loc.gov/2023035509

Published by Nova Science Publishers, Inc. † New York

I thank my dear wife, Kubra Bulbul, who has always supported me.

Emre Bulbul

Contents

Preface

Cardiovascular applications with a tissue engineering approach in tissue damage treatments lead the way regarding clinical applications. Designing the optimal and functional vascular network will be essential for repairing congenital heart anomalies and treating heart valve diseases or ischemic heart disease.

Many diseases have genetic properties. For this reason, we are investigating more about genetics. For example, genetic diagnostic methods and therapies have recently become an undeniable part of cancer treatment. Increasing knowledge of genetic control of vascular development opens new paths for developing the most challenging medical treatments. New studies are rapidly increasing nowadays to understand unknown paths of this control.

Regenerative therapies can solve vascular problems in erectile dysfunction thanks to their neovascularization effects. Using autologous bioengineered materials in treatments may be more advantageous than synthetic materials in foreign body reactions. In addition, bioengineering technology products can be edited, and they can improve the efficacy and safety of treatments. Both regenerative therapy and tissue engineering can be applied as a component of minimally invasive treatments in treating urethral strictures. Tissue-engineering techniques can also be used in penile length augmentation surgery. However, prospective studies in larger patient groups are needed for the efficacy and safety of regenerative therapies and tissue-engineering methods.

Chapter 1-Establishing effective vascularized networks in engineered tissues and organs is the greatest strategic challenge in tissue engineering. Biomolecules have emerged as a possible contender for inducing vascularization and angiogenesis, resulting in effective tissue repair due to numerous research and technological developments.

Chapter 2- Since tissue repair is essential in increasing the survival of the biomaterial in tissue engineering, where new steps are taken in the production of biomaterials in the repair and regeneration of damaged tissues and failed organs, all factors and diseases that impair oxygenation and perfusion will lead the tissue to failure. All conditions that may cause hypoxemia and prevent angiogenesis should be investigated in patients. Oxygen support therapy and hyperbaric oxygen therapy can increase the success rate. The use of oxygen-producing tissue-engineered biomaterials, believed to be beneficial in preventing problems of oxygen diffusion in large tissue implants, should be evaluated in these patients.

Chapter 3- Knowledge of genetics and its role in diseases is rapidly increasing. Chronic diseases, cardiovascular pathologies, and cancer have a strong genetic background. A thorough understanding of the role of genetics opens up new possibilities for the prevention and treatment of these conditions. One stepstone of this understanding is the genetic pathways of vascular development and their effect on disease progression. Strict genetic paths control vasculogenesis and angiogenesis. Initially, these processes were believed to occur only in embryonic life; however, recent studies showed they also occur in adult tissues. The continuation of vascular development in adult tissues shows that vascularization can effectively treat chronic diseases. This chapter will try to explain the genetic control of vascular development in both embryonal and adult life and discuss new tools for diagnosing, preventing, and treating diseases in light of the knowledge of these processes.

Chapter 4- Tissue vascularisation can be impaired in many infectious diseases. For example, microvascular thrombosis can occur in many infectious diseases causing sepsis. It plays an essential role in multiple organ failures and mortality. In COVID-19, endothelial damage occurs through direct and indirect mechanisms. Cytokines, complement activation, activated platelets, and immune cells play a role in indirect damage. The development of targeted therapies will guide the treatment of not only COVID-19 but also many other viral and bacterial infections.

Chapter 5- Sepsis; It causes health professionals to experience economic and medical problems in managing the disease, as both mortality and morbidity rates are high and hospital infections are common. Entry of the SARS-CoV-2 virus into the human body is most commonly via droplet to the upper respiratory tract. It enters the host cell by using angiotensin-converting enzyme 2 (ACE-2) receptors, which are found at high rates in the lung's alveoli, myocyte cells of the heart, vascular endothelial cells, and many cells. This virus has a high affinity for the host cell; it is known to act by using the ACE-2 receptor and binding with its spike protein. The SARS-CoV-2 virus has a high affinity for ACE-2, especially in alveolar epithelial type II and endothelial cells. The virus has been shown to attack and damage these cells directly. SARS-CoV-2 uses virus spike protein and binds to the ACE-2 receptor, injuring alveolar vascular epithelial cells, macrophages, and monocytes. Many studies have examined and tried to define the mechanisms of coagulopathy developing due to COVID-19 sepsis. However, the existing mechanisms have been insufficient to explain the coagulopathy that occurs. Unfortunately, the treatment strategies related to these did not give satisfactory results. Although we did not leave it behind ultimately, we left the moderate and severe COVID-19 disease behind at the time I wrote the chapter. However, we may encounter different pandemics in the future. We must be prepared to eliminate such epidemics with the least damage.

Chapter 6- To understand the normal functions of vascular cells and how they are affected by various vascular movements, researchers and clinicians need to treat patients with peripheral artery disease, coronary artery disease, and hypertension. It is, therefore, essential to know the basic concepts of vascular diseases and to learn how common diseases change the foundations of vascular control. This chapter will provide an overview of the basic concepts of cardiovascular diseases.

Chapter 7- The endothelium is an excellent barrier between the circulating blood and the vessel wall. It is considered the largest endocrine organ in the body, with the molecules it secretes and its receptors. The smooth functioning of the endothelium's special functions is essential for the perfect functioning of human physiology. Endothelial functions are essential in the physiopathology and treatment of musculoskeletal diseases. In addition, endothelial damage is the main problem in the pathology of diseases in many areas, such as muscle-tendon injuries, enthesitis, tendinopathies, fracture healing, and cartilage problems. In many treatments, such as fracture healing, therapy of tendinopathies, and repair of cartilage defects, the goal should be to help vascular functions work correctly and to improve endothelin functions for tissue healing. A better understanding of musculoskeletal diseases has led us to seek both the source of the problem and the solution at the endothelial level.

Chapter 8- Many treatment methods are being developed in modern medicine with innovative approaches. For example, regenerative therapies and tissue engineering are used in many fields of medicine. Regenerative therapies are a prevalent research topic today. Treatments such as stem cell therapy and platelet-rich plasma are among the vascular-regenerative treatments. Regenerative therapies are tried in urology practice, especially in erectile dysfunction, where vascular pathology is common. At the same time, it is used for urethral stricture disease, in which damaged urethral tissue heal with fibrosis. Regenerative therapies can solve vascular problems in erectile dysfunction thanks to their neovascularization effects. Both regenerative therapy and tissue engineering can be applied as a component of minimally invasive treatments in treating urethral strictures. In addition, some studies continue to reduce the contraction of bioengineered graft materials in cell cultures.

Chapter 1

Biomolecules for Triggering Vascularization in Soft and Hard Tissue Healing

Pratik Das[1,*]
Sonali Jana[2,*]
Piyali Basak[1]
Biswanath Kundu[3]
and Samit Kumar Nandi[2†]
[1]School of Bioscience & Engineering, Jadavpur University, Kolkata, India
[2]West Bengal University of Animal & Fishery Sciences, Kshudiram Bose Sarani, Kolkata, India
[3]Bioceramics and Coating Division, CSIR-Central Glass and Ceramic Research Institute, Kolkata, India

Abstract

Establishing effective vascularized networks in engineered tissues and organs is the greatest strategic challenge in tissue engineering. Biomolecules have emerged as a possible contender for inducing vascularization and angiogenesis, resulting in effective tissue repair due to numerous research and technological developments. Extracellular growth factors, cytokines, peptides, proteins, and signaling peptides are essential in defining and regulating various cellular actions. Complex biomolecules like oligosaccharides and carbohydrates are gaining prominence in tissue healing applications. Naturally produced biomolecules have a significant role in initiating angiogenesis and

* Equally contributed and joint first author.
† Corresponding Author's Email: samitnandi1967@gmail.com.

In: Vascularization and Its Role in Medicine and Tissue Engineering
Editors: Emre Bulbul and Murat Oguz Ozilhan
ISBN: 979-8-89113-041-8

fostering efficient vascularization. Diverse and complex phytochemicals derived from plant sources can also stimulate vascularization in tissue engineering. An effective report summarizes the influence of the important biomolecules on increasing vascularization in soft and hard tissue healing. Consequently, this chapter outlines the features and capabilities of various biomolecules and their impact on supporting efficient vascularization in tissue repair. This chapter will try to provide an overview of the accomplishments and drawbacks of the current scientific methodologies.

Keywords: endothelium, endothelial dysfunction, tissue healing, tissue engineering, scaffolds

Introduction

To perform all the basic functionalities of life, a human body consists of billions of microscopic parts that work together in an organized manner. This system comprises billions of such parts that have their own identity and exist in various forms. The first and foremost is the cell. Our life started as a cell. The journey to this elaborate system of human bodies began as a cell. It is a fundamental structural and functional unit of energy that resembles a brick building block of huge mansions. One can deny everything except that cells are the simplest unit of life that can reproduce and exist independently. Cells define tissues as an organization of similar cells with different kinds and levels of intercellular substances. In the realm of tissue engineering, further injuries can be identified. The study of tissue engineering uses the creation of biological alternatives to maintain, repair, and enhance the tissue structures in our bodies [1].

The ineffective treatment of wounds greatly hampers human health. The financial and social expenses for healthcare organizations, professionals, patients, and their families grow when a patient doesn't heal or takes longer than expected. Inadequate wound care could cause bleeding, infections, inflammation, scarring, and difficulty with angiogenesis and regeneration, among other issues. According to the World Health Organization estimations, about 3/4th of the world's population relies on traditional treatments and medical herbs for basic healthcare, and 85% of this population relies on only plants for medicine [2].

Some of the specific tissue injuries are soft and hard tissue injuries. Soft tissue injuries are when the skin has been cut open with blisters, cuts, etc. On the other hand, closed soft tissue injuries occur beneath the skin and involve no external bleeding, unlike open wounds. This includes bruising, pulls, sprains, and strains [3]. Moving onto the hard tissue injuries, these deal with cracks or breaks within bones that further lead to bruising, swelling, or fracture. Be it injuries related to epidermal tissue or the ones involving skeletal muscles; both require vascularization techniques to heal. Vascularization is a process in which the angioblast cells differentiate into endothelial cells to form primitive vascular networks that help transport blood, oxygen, and nutrients to tissue at the microvascular interface. Modern vascularization technology allows multidisciplinary approaches to include engineered biomolecule cells and angiogenic factors that regulate therapeutic wound healing and initiate tissue regeneration and repair [4].

Coming to angiogenesis, cytokines and growth factors [5] play an important role in tissue regeneration and the tissue healing process [6]. Proangiogenic, GF's, and cytokines are included in the biomolecules that regulate distinctive signaling pathways to automate tissue engineering regenerative approaches. These macromolecular cells are frequently released by endothelial cells, smooth muscle cells, fibroblasts, inflammatory cells, and platelets. When these macromolecular cells attach to their transmembrane receptors on cells, they signal various downstream angiogenic pathways. Some of the most important pro-angiogenic cytokines and factors include MAPK (mitogen-activated protein), bfGf (basic fibroblast growth factor), and VEGF (vascular endothelial growth factor) [7].

The removal of pathogenic microorganisms is known as inflammation, a normal and primary component of the wound-healing process. However, incomplete microbial removal occurs because of the absence of successful cleaning [8]. Inflammation may persist for a longer time if wounds of any kind remain unclean for quite a time. Moreover, the inflammatory process will be prolonged if pro-inflammatory cytokines like interleukin-1 (IL-1) and TNF-alpha are used to sustain it. Such cytokines are responsible for supporting bacteria and endotoxins, which might worsen the wound healing process [9]. If this continues, the wound can become chronic and stop healing. Matrix metalloproteinases (MMPs), a class of proteases, break down the ECM and are produced in greater amounts due to prolonged inflammation. Together with the elevated protease content, there is a decrease in the levels of the naturally occurring protease inhibitors.

Different Classes of Biomolecules and Their Properties

As we discussed before how biomolecules play an interesting role in vascularization and tissue repair or regeneration, let us know more about these from the very basics.

Nearly 300 trillion cells are equipped to systemize the human body and carry out its basic life processes. The biomolecular and organic compounds compulsively help cells in carrying out fundamental functions. These are usually involved in various life functions and exist in multiple forms and sizes. The major types of these biomolecular include primary elements like carbon, phosphorus, sulfur, and hydrogen.

Carbohydrates

The element carbon is the major involvement in forming biomolecules [10], which combine with other elements to create carbon derivatives. Four major classes of such molecules are formed after the polymerization of their monomeric units. It is necessary to have plenty of carbohydrates in your diet because it is essential in forming molecules like polyhydroxy acetone or polyhydroxy ketone. Thus, it supplies a lot of energy for our bodies. The most abundant biomolecules on earth are carbohydrates which can be sub-categorized based on the number of products they form during hydrolysis.

Monosaccharides

Foremost are monosaccharides or single units of a carbohydrate chain. The polyhydroxy aldehyde or polyhydroxy ketones comprise a single unit of this polysaccharide. They are an entirely crystalline colorless substance that is completely hydrolyzed in water and is involved in the body's energy production processes. Glucose, ribose, arabinose, and arabinose are all that can be compiled into this list [11].

Disaccharides

Moving onto the next category of disaccharides, they comprise two monomeric sugar units connected with o- glycosidic linkage. Some examples are sucrose and lactose. Besides, which are composed of more than two sugar units are known as polysaccharides; also known by the term 'glycine,' they come into two categories; lipopolysaccharide and heteropolysaccharides [12].

Lipopolysaccharide

Lipopolysaccharide or homopolysaccharide includes one kind or form of many monomeric units joined together [13]. Thanks to its various functions, it can further be categorized into structural and storage homopolysaccharides. Chitin and cellulose are examples of structural lipopolysaccharide, while starch, glycogen, and insulin are some organic compounds that can be mentioned under the storage lipopolysaccharide [14, 15].

Heteropolysaccharides

Another sub-category of polysaccharides is heteropolysaccharides which contain two or more different sugar units, which form one polymeric team. These play different roles as they are found within the bacterial cell wall providing structural function and heparin that acts as an anticoagulant in blood clotting [16].

Proteins

Protein, the second biomolecular, consists of unbranched polymers of amino acid residues. There are, in total, 22 amino acids that vary in function and location. Based on their structural formation, proteins are categorized into primary, secondary, and tertiary structures. The primary structure is formed when two amino acid peptides join together. The secondary structure is created due to hydrogen bonds amid the amide hydrogen and the carbonyl oxygen of the peptide backbone. It is in the form of a folded structure like alpha and beta structures. The last structure is a three-dimensional conformation of the side chains that makes up proteins and another important amino acid in our body. The tertiary structure is made of two or unique. Various bonds are present between these structures like hydrophobic, electrostatic, hydrogen, and covalent bonds. The formed quaternary structure is a result of multiple subunits. Protein is one of the most integral biological components for the proper functioning of our body. Processes such as DNA replication, cell signaling, formation of cells, tissue regeneration along with various metabolic reactions are carried out by protein. [17]

Nucleic Acids

Nucleic acids are macromolecules present in both viruses and cells and are an integral part of the cell that trespasses the transmission of genetic information and its storage. The nucleic acid is composed of three components: A nitrogenous base, five carbon sugars, and phosphonic acid or nucleic acid that exists in two forms DNA and RNA. DNA is the genetic structure inside the nucleus acid that exists in two states as the hereditary system inside the nucleus controls all the cell's activities [18, 19]. Conversely, RNA acts as both genetic material and performs enzymatic catalyzation. The various types of RNA are tRNA, mRNA, and rRNA. If we compose the functions of RNA and DNA, it is very tough to leverage them on their importance [20].

Lipids

So far, we have covered several aspects of biomolecules. Biomolecules help organisms to develop, endure and procreate. They interact with one another to carry out biochemical reactions to sustain life. These reactions are studied in detail in biochemistry.

The fourth, biochemical macromolecules, are either insoluble or partially soluble lipids in water or other organic solvents [21]. They are hydrophobic and structurally form membranous structures like glycolipids, steroids, eicosanoids, and some plasma lipoprotein that varies according to density. Let us know in detail about them:

Fatty Acids

The simplest form of lipids is composed of 4-36 carbon hydrocarbon chains and an acidic group. They can be present in varied conditions. Some are linear, while some seem to be branched [22].

Waxes

t exists in the form of an organization of esters, long-chain alcohols, and fatty acids. They are composed of hydrocarbon chains of up to 14-36 carbon. The best available quality of wax is palmitic acid and triacontanol alcohol [23].

Phospholipids

These comprise phosphate, alcohol connected to phosphate, fatty acids, and a platform for attaching fatty acids. They are a component of the organisms' cell membrane.

Steroids

These lipids have saccharide groups in them. They participate in signal transduction and are parts of the cell membrane.

Eicosanoids

They are produced by polyunsaturated fatty acids, which contain 20 carbons. They carry out several tasks. Leukotrienes play a role in inflammation and chemotaxis; prostaglandins stimulate uterine contraction and lower blood pressure; thromboxane operate as vasoconstrictors and promote platelet aggregation.

Need and Challenges for Hard and Soft Tissue Healing

Tissue healing is a complex and coordinated event requiring the urgent and necessary participation of various cellular populations, soluble mediators and the underlying matrix stage whereupon these complex events culminate in tissue building to restore the functions and repair the damaged tissue concerned. In the face of the challenge whereby tissue is so severely impaired both functionally and structurally by chronicity, cancer, severe trauma, or an anomaly of congenital nature; conventional therapeutics will least serve the intended purpose. Thus, resorting to organ transplantation is often the first choice. However, it too suffers from several flaws; the demand and supply of organs are often mismatched, have biocompatibility issues, and are susceptible to immune rejection. With the advancement in technologies, the biomedical sector has seen a renaissance of innovations that has equipped humans with innumerable therapeutics for damaged tissues. With the emergence of advanced biomaterials, the tissue engineering field to has developed rapidly. It utilizes cells, scaffolds, and growth factors to regenerate the lost tissues and organs. Various synthetic and natural polymers are being investigated for the development of scaffolds. Natural polymers such as collagen, chitosan, alginate, and gelatin are some of the promising raw materials for the development of constructs for tissue engineering. The challenges and goals of tissue engineering are very certain in that it focuses on the generation of therapeutics for the cure of ailments/ diseases that are almost impossible to be achieved by the existing remedies [24]. The use of varied growth factors and cells has been extensively investigated in the field of tissue engineering in recent times. Another important challenge faced in the regeneration of both hard and soft tissues is inadequate vascularization which greatly hampers efficient tissue healing. Cell seeded 3D scaffold implants known for potential in bone tissue regeneration have been associated with the major drawback of implant failure from the inability to generate adequate microvasculature in the host. The spontaneous capillary network developed during implantation is known to regress within a short time thus restricting the healing process. The poor vascular supply at the implant site further restricts the ability of the tissues to flush out the degradation products and be replenished with adequate nutrients and oxygen. The accumulation of by-products of metabolism instigates inflammatory responses which further negatively affects the healing. The process that intends to establish a connection between the implant and host circulation is termed inosculation or anastomosis [25]. While this needs time and a conducive intraosseous microenvironment the challenges lie in developing more advanced strategies for enhanced neovascularization.

Protein, Growth Factors and Peptides in Tissue Healing

Various proteins, growth factors, and peptides are utilized in tissue regeneration and repair processes; protein hydrolysates provide a rich source of protein required during tissue repair and damage. Protein hydrolysates are useful in tissue repair because they allow for more amino acids than whole proteins or some peptides. They help provide a strong insulinogenic effect that regulates protein and enhances the structure of muscles with the help of branched-chain amino acids. If utilized in our body, it contributes to the healing of tissues caused by surgery, ulcers, burns, and muscle-damaging exercise [26].

Another substitute that is quite helpful in the tissue healing process is the growth factor. Growth factors are molecules that stimulate processes like differentiation, migration, proliferation, and morphogenesis in our ills. Gfs have given rise to a great deal of hope for a regenerative medicine strategy because such a mechanism is necessary for tissue development and healing. GF-based therapies [27]are now scarce despite their benefits for tissue repair in combat; this is because it takes many administrations and doses to maintain an effective concentration, which is quite expensive. Furthermore, supraphysiological doses may have negative side effects and be useless. Peptides are the third most essential constituents that help in tissue repair. These are a basic sequence of amino acids, which are the special building blocks of protein. One of the ways it helps our body is by wound healing. Certain peptides are responsible of producing a glue-like substance that binds cells together as in connective tissue. This gluey substance is only collagen produced by special repair cells to reverse tissue injury. This particulate material is highly useful in connective tissue growth and beneficial in healing connective tissue injuries like tendonitis, some tendon tears, and ruptures [28]. Some of the most important examples of peptides are BPC-157, TB-500, and CJC-1295; these sought to have incredibly done wonders in the prospect of tissue regeneration and repairs [29].

People who are aging must realize that with age, there is a rapid decline in the growth hormone and other hormones, which has a lot to do with the pace of tissue maintenance and repair. The rate of tissue injury healing can also be controlled with the growth hormone, secretagogues, and several other peptides.

Other peptides involved in the growth process are thymosin beta 4, MGF, IGF-1, and CJC-1295/IPAMORELIN [30, 31]. Talking about these inducers, they help to get a jump on rapid tissue regeneration and healing.

- Thymosin Beta 4 promotes blood vessel, muscle cells, and skin cell regeneration, thus helping in the regeneration process as fast as possible. Stimulated from the thymus gland, it helps in the faster recovery of damaged tissue [32].

- MGF or Mechano growth factor is essential for recovery, repair, and growth of new cells by causing muscle cells to split and develop as two, thus becoming a potent inducer of muscle growth [33].
- IGF-1 is another important growth factor that our bodies produce and thus, provides a great enhancement for muscle building [34].
- CJC-1295 or ipamorelin combination has an effective and strong effect on the release of GH, IGF-5, and certain peptides like collagen, thus helping cellular repair and conditional tissue regeneration [35].

Natural Biomolecules and Phytochemicals in Tissue Healing

Phytochemicals and biochemicals are bioactive [27] nutritional plant remedial chemicals that might offer effective and advantageous health benefits and minimize chronic diseases. They are found in fruits, cereals, vegetables, and other plant foods. They positively impact human health with several substantial health advantages. Besides, phytochemicals have a high antioxidant potential and are significantly important. Phytochemicals include phytoestrogens, flavonoids, isoflavonoids, polyphenols, anthocyanidins, terpenoids, carotenoids, limonoids, phytosterols, glucosinolates, etc. Phytochemicals may affect human health and illness risk at the community level due to their increasing prevalence in the diet and apparent low toxicity. They are also available in the form of dietary phytochemicals. Dietary phytochemicals can be grouped into two categories based on their bioavailability: lipid-soluble, including phenolics and polyphenols, and water-soluble, including carotenoids, tocochromanols, and curcuminoids.

Phytochemicals [36] or biological chemicals have shown considerable response in preventing and treating microbial infections and wounds, blood clotting, infection prevention, and tissue repair. They promote clotting, combat infection, and accelerate wound healing. It is said that polyphenol-rich medicinal herbs have remarkable wound healing processes. Phenolic astringent, antibacterial, and free radical scavenging abilities are the key reasons they help heal wounds. The potential of polyphenol substances, including flavonoids, enhance wound healing primarily due to their antibacterial and antioxidant activities. By reducing lipid peroxidation, they also help to prevent cell damage and increase the vitality of collagen fibrils. Many still use such conventional wound treatment and tissue regeneration methods in less developed nations. Despite significant advancements in synthetic drug chemistry and antibiotics, plants play an important role in medicine's traditional and modern systems.

Herbal medication and meals made from plants have emerged as alternatives, even in highly developed nations, as people have become aware of the hazardous effects of synthetic pharmaceuticals. The current medical system makes use of both traditional medicinal herbs and their pharmaceutical formulations as folk medicines [37]. It is possible to treat and cure diseases including ulcers, wound healing, skin infections, inflammation, scabies, leprosy, and venereal illness with herbal remedies. Herbal remedies clean wounds, remove dead tissue, and provide a moist environment that encourages the emergence of an ideal natural healing climate. Many plants are used in folklore cultures to cure burns, wounds, and cuts; some of them are mentioned in great detail below:

Centella asiatica

This herb, used to speed up wound healing, was also known as Asian pennywort. Extracts from the aerial sections of the *Centella asiatica* are reported to help with the recovery of chronic ulcers in terms of size, depth, and location. To prove its additional and exemplary values, a punch-type wound has been found to improve from the effects of asiaticoside, a compound isolated from *Centella asiatica* [38].

Curcumin

Curcumin is an active ingredient found in the *Curcuma longa* root, and a member of the ginger family has been used for medical purposes and as a food flavor for many years. Practitioners of traditional Ayurvedic medicine use curcumin to treat skin injuries, liver ailments, respiratory illnesses, and diabetes [39]. One of the most well-researched nutraceuticals, curcumin has been utilized often by several ethnic groups for decades. It has been demonstrated that a highly pleiotropic molecule interacts with important biological pathways at the transcription, translation, and post-translational stages, Also In several of the target pathways, NF-yB, pro-inflammatory cytokines, apoptosis, cyclooxygenase 2, 5-LOX, STAT3, C-reactive protein, cell adhesion molecules, and prostaglandin E2. Besides this, curcumin also promotes fibroblast proliferation, granulation tissue growth, and collagen deposition in the healing of cutaneous wounds [40].

Panax ginseng

One of the many bioactive substances found in *Panax ginseng* is from a family of saponins, which is the most potent active component (called ginsenosides by Russian researchers and panaxosides by Asian scientists). It has been demonstrated that Panax ginseng root extracts can greatly speed up the healing process after laser burns and excisional wound injuries while also shielding the skin from acute UVB irradiation. According to studies, Panax ginseng extracts boost human dermal fibroblasts' ability to increase, promote keratinocyte migration, and produce collagen in vitro [41]. It has also been demonstrated that ginsenoside Rb2 is isolated from Panax ginseng, which stimulates the production of fibronectin and the receptor, keratin and collagenase I, as well as epidermal growth factor and receptor, for the development of epidermis in raft culture [42].

Many other medicinal plants like Neem, German chamomile, and Budock are also available that provide dietary bioactive materials that help tissue regeneration, repair, and healing. Researchers are looking at new mixtures, bandages, and medicinal plant components to create a more affordable, effective, stable, and provides long-lasting delivery system for the control, management, and treatment of wounds. The availability of innovative materials and the emergence of nanotechnology have improved wound treatment and made it more patient-focused [43]. The cutting-edge view of technology for creating wound healing systems incorporates tissue engineering and regenerative medicine. New research avenues in wound care management will be made possible by improved quality control methods for identifying, screening, and measuring herbal components, as well as by well-designed pre-clinical and clinical trials.

Oligosaccharides and Carbohydrates in Tissue Healing

The management of wounds has witnessed significant advancement over the years. From protective wound dressings in the earlier times which were meant to protect from external damaging agents to more advanced grafts/dressings that tend to regenerate the wound bed with less scarring. Several carbohydrates have been recognized that stimulate various stages of wound healing and thereby they are being continuously investigated. A wide range of carbohydrates such as polysaccharides and oligosaccharides such as dextran, cellulose, (1–3)-b-d –glucans, chitin, chitosan, alginic acid/ alginate, hyaluronic acid, and sulfated polysaccharides have shown promising outcomes in tissue healing. Polysaccharides are bestowed with unique characteristics which render them suitable for tissue healing applications. They are biocompatible, biodegradable, and have low cytotoxicity. With varied functional groups these function in carrying bioactive molecules with antimicrobial properties. Thus, these are endowed with distinct tissue healing and reconstruction abilities [44]. Stimulation of angiogenic activity within the healing wound bed is crucial to efficient tissue regeneration which otherwise would turn chronic with persistent inflammation and infection. Cellulose nanocrystals have been shown to stimulate vascularization along with promoting cellular functions such as cell migration and proliferation, particularly in the liquid crystalline phase. So multifunctional injectable hydrogels based on cellulose were developed containing catechol and Ag. These hydrogels stimulated neovascularization, had antibacterial effects, and showed potential for efficient tissue regeneration [45]. In the repair of full-thickness skin wounds, a multifunctional wound dressing composed of alginate/chitosan/fucoidan (ACF) sponges remarkably promoted the healing of full-thickness skin wounds by upregulating the expression of angiogenic marker CD 31, along with enhancing epithelialization, collagen deposition, hemostatic and antibacterial effects [46]. The oligosaccharide that has been expansively investigated in wound healing for several intrinsic benefits is oligosaccharides of Hyaluronan/hyaluronic acid. They can stimulate angiogenesis during wound healing by a signal transduction pathway whereby the Hyaluronan oligosaccharides (o-HA) bind to the (RHAMM) Receptor for HA-Mediated Motility thereby mediating the proliferation of endothelial cells [47]. O-HA is observed to modulate several key phenomena during the regenerative process of healing. The ECM matrix responds to o-HA treatment by enhanced collagen and granulation tissue deposition, and proliferation of fibroblasts with upregulated expressions for cytokines that aid in granulation tissue deposition. A marked increase in neovascularization and lymph vessels is also evident resulting in efficient wound healing [48]. Wang et al. (2016) suggested that under hyperglycemic conditions O-HA is capable of stimulating angiogenesis in wounds by enhanced expression of TGF beta1 and phosphorylation of Src and ERK (extracellular signal-related kinases) [49]. Chitosan oligosaccharides-based nanofiber also shows promising effects on wound healing through the regulation of early stages of healing mediated via the TGFβ1/Smad signaling pathway involving the upregulation of a multitude of cytokines regulating the healing pathways [50]. Recent approaches toward enhancing vascularization in healing tissues are the fabrication of vascularized constructs through advanced (3D) bioprinting technology. For wound care, a novel bioprinted gelatin methacryloyl (GelMA) shell containing cell was constructed over a cell-laden core consisting of peptide-functionalized, succinylated chitosan/dextran aldehyde. This designed construct with specialized molecules having revascularizing ability was observed to promote the growth of human bone-marrow-derived mesenchymal stem cells and human umbilical vein endothelial cells. Microvasularization and enhanced wound healing was achieved through *in vitro* studies thereby establishing the potential of such advanced methodologies in the future generation of revascularized tissues [51].

Nucleic Acids (NAs) in Healing

Nucleic acids (NAs) including small-interfering RNA (siRNA), microRNA (miRNA), plasmid DNA (pDNA), aptamers, and antisense oligonucleotides (ASOs) have recently been the focus of extensive study, leading to the creation of a novel therapeutic approach for wound healing. In this context, several NA delivery strategies, including dendrimers, scaffolds, lipid nanoparticles, polymeric nanoparticles, hydrogels, and metal nanoparticles, have been investigated [52]. However, there is still a significant obstacle presented by NA's potential for translation. Thus, various NAs must be distinguished, and the best means of dispersal for them must be determined. NAs are among the most effective tools for altering cellular biology. After several failed attempts in the 1990s, scientists have found that a NA multi-functional architecture may regulate the release of physiologically active components, speeding the healing of wounds by increasing the dermis' natural ability to repair itself. Scaffold-mediated release of DNA and RNA-based products can also repress genes responsible for chronic wounds, opening the door to novel regenerative medicine approaches. Reportedly, tFNAs can promote the growth and migration of HaCaTs, HDFs, and HUVECs in a high-glucose setting. Accelerating epithelialization, vascularization, collagen synthesis, and growth factor secretion via the Wnt pathway, tFNAs can hasten the healing of diabetic wounds [53]. Gene targeting in vitro and in vivo can improve angiogenic and osteogenic differentiation capacity, however, miRNAs can degrade in the acidic endo-/lysosome and stimulate the intracellular release of miRNAs [54]. The therapeutic application of biomaterials for the administration of NAs to promote skin wound healing is still in its infancy, and many challenges remain. In general, the next generation of platforms for NA administration in wound healing will need to be nontoxic, have "stealth" qualities to prevent macrophage infiltration and immunological reactivity, have strong pharmacokinetic properties, and be able to target particular tissues [55]. Furthermore, the limits of localized growth factor delivery can be avoided by the use of tissue-engineered platform-mediated gene therapies. Additionally, many types of NAs and pharmaceuticals might be applied to a single gauze to synergistically stimulate angiogenesis, activate macrophage aggregation, and promote cell migration and re-epithelialization. Also essential are distribution networks that can rush the right medicines to patients when they need them [56].

Discussion and Future Perspectives

Sophisticated strategies are currently being researched under investigation to ensure rapid blood and biological constituents towards tissues. Their methods involve the stimulation of blood vessel formation and the generation of formed microvascular networks regarding vascularization. Such research highlights the importance of vascularization and various approaches in regenerative and multiple systems in regenerative medicine and tissue engineering.

Weinberg and Berg's considerable advancement in fabrication in 1986 created the first blood vessels from collagen, smooth muscle cells, fibroblast, and endothelial cells. Since this development, there has been a synergistic combination of advanced fabrication methods with biomaterials formulation and vascular tissue development. Many newer technologies like nanotechnology, 3D bioprinting technology, and dynamic maturation systems like bioreactors have led to the advancement of vascular tissue engineering.

Moreover, new formulas, dressings, and compositions of bioactive materials are being explored, which will create a full-fledged efficient, cost-effective, stable, and sustainable delivery system for the treatment and management of wounds. Such research has been aligned around therapeutic methods due to advancements in the acute and chronic wound treatment spectrum of medicine like Ayurveda. Tissue engineering and newer regenerative methods, including novel methods like nanotechnology and screening processes for quantifying herbal components, are developing for a better-seeking future. Many studies regarding well-designed pre-clinical and clinical studies are undertaken, which would open newer ways for research in wound care management.

The healing of wounds is a complicated and multicellular operation preserved throughout evolution to restore the skin's barrier. Multiple cell types collaborate to complete this process, together with endothelial cells, fibroblasts [5] keratinocytes, and platelets. These relocation, penetration, accretion, and separation of cells w result in a swelling response, and the growth of newer tissues, with eventually the healing of the wound. An equally complicated signaling network of multiple growth factors, cytokines, and chemokines drives and controls this intricate process. Mentioned below are several important growth factors:

- Interleukin (IL)
- platelet-derived growth factor (PDGF)
- transforming growth factor beta (TGF-beta)
- Connective tissue growth factor (CTGF)
- granulocyte-macrophage colony-stimulating factor (GM-CSF)
- Fibroblast growth factor (FGF)
- Tumor necrosis factor (TNF)

Infection usually occurs when a pathogen like bacteria, fungi, or some other organisms tries to enter the wound and disrupt the process of healing. If the wound is infected with some faulty bodies, it might take a lot of time to heal. This happens because then the body's energy is utilized in protecting and cleaning the wound instead of healing it. Therefore, with this, it cannot reach the regeneration stage properly.

According to the previous reports, it can be highlighted that angiogenesis and vascularization are the primary and most effective methods for boosting tissue regeneration and repair. Various constituents like growth factors, proteases, and peptides provide inherent benefits depending on the target tissues. To speed up the vascularization process, selecting biomaterials, biomolecules and bio-active chemicals that direct the mass of cells is crucial. Choosing carriers and scaffolds [57] that trespass cells toward the microvascular network are important to heal wounds using multiple growth factors and genetic manipulation.

Phytochemicals, as we discussed earlier, have the potential to regenerate tissue and are considered untapped "treasure homes." Ayurveda uses indigenous, affordable, non-toxic formulations of phytochemicals in tissue engineering techniques, which combines conventional wisdom with cutting-edge technology. The creation of phytochemical-incorporated tissue-engineered scaffolds may be accomplished using advanced methods like nanotechnology and electrospinning [58].

In the United States, there seem to be over 6.5 million people with wounds that don't heal properly. There are various causes of improper wound healing. How you heal can change as you grow. Wounds may heal more slowly in elderly persons. Poor blood flow may be caused by several medical problems. Many other circumstances can lead to insufficient wound healing with causes like diabetes or obesity, hypertension, and Vascular illness.

Wound healing [59] is a collaboratively intensive process that involves allergic reactions, propagation, and remodeling as its three parallel steps assist tissue regeneration. A proliferative process is a repair response triggered by the inflammatory process [60], and it is further defined by vascular responses such as hemostasis and coagulation of blood. Examples of cellular activities are the takeover of white blood cells and the release of antibiotics and cytokines. The epithelium is created during the proliferative process to cover the wound surface, and granulation tissue then grows to fill the wound area. To produce granulation tissue, fibroblasts multiply, collagen [61] and other extracellular matrices are deposited, and new blood vessels are formed. The remodeling process returns the tissue's structural integrity and functional competency when the new tissue develops inside the wound. Having covered the four wound healing stages, let us understand the clinical significance of wound healing. Any disruption or change in the process of wound healing leads to excessive wound or chronic wound formation the paths followed by excessive wound formation and the pants followed by excessive wound healing are not normalized. This can be a result of continuous localized inflammation and lead to extreme collagen syntheses, Exaggerated EEM concentrations like keloid and hypertrophic scars.

A chronic wound can be defined as one which takes up to 4 weeks for healing. Several factors that lead to chronic wound formation are age, radiation, insufficient oxygenation and perfusion, malnutrition, etc. Support surfaces, friction, and shear or effective repositioning are some of the extrinsic factors. Several other local factors like moisture, faulty wound closure, entering of foreign bodies, and ischemia can also be included in the list. [62]

Since Yuan Cheng Fung first coined the word "tissue engineering" [63] in 1985, when only a few selective cartilage, skin, artificial tissues, and bladder, successfully made the transition to clinical use.

But before they can be sold, other, more complicated organs need a lot of development. Research in the field of bone and tissue engineering has been centered on osteoconductivity, osteoblasts, biomaterial creation, and the establishment of fabrication techniques for the past 30 years [32]. The significance of the development of a functional bone vascular network, however, has necessitated more focus. Recently, there has been a noticeable change in the direction of bone vascular creation research in the field of bone tissue engineering. There is no longer any question that functional vasculature is essential to the effective clinical outcomes of engineered tissue constructs. For an implant to survive and integrate, oxygen, nutrients, and metabolic waste must be removed through a vascular network in bone.

However, the three stages of damaged healing tissues [61]are not straightforward and time-limited processes. Burns, serious wounds, and surgical wounds are examples of acute wounds, which are wounds that heal quickly. A clean, uninfected, and incisional wound that has been approximated to be a surgical injury [64] illustrates a normal acute wound. While the formation of new tissues with similar structure and functions to the retained skin is the intended result of organized healing, regeneration is uncommon. When tissues are properly cured, a product that is physically and functionally acceptable but not identical is formed. The release of different GFs and cytokines [65] at the affected site regulates wound healing.

Conclusion

Tissue healing can is significantly hampered by ineffective neovascularization at the site of the defect resulting in poor clinical outcomes. Fabrication of biomaterial-based scaffolds with adequate vascularizing abilities is the prevailing challenge that has drawn considerable attention from the scientific community. The decisive roles of vascularized biomaterials as bone, and skin substitutes and in various soft and hard tissue engineering have been investigated widely. Biological molecules such as growth factors, cytokines, proteins, and carbohydrates to plant-derived phytochemicals have served promising roles as vascularizing agents in tissue scaffolds. While the syncing between angiogenesis and osteogenesis is an essential prerequisite to the restoration of the bony defect; in soft tissues, angiogenesis – granulation tissue and matrix remodeling serve a similar purpose in soft tissue restoration. Cell-based and scaffold encapsulating bioactive molecules-based approaches are essential means of developing efficient angiogenesis in tissue defects. To fulfill the necessity of an optimum long-term vascularizing scaffold, it should essentially be economic, controlled, and reproducible. While a lot has been achieved towards acknowledging newer molecules with vascularizing abilities; there is yet a broad gap wherein we need to develop *in vitro* vascularized implants as well as tissues and organs with the advanced technologies and knowledge at our disposal.

Acknowledgments

The authors are thankful to the Science and Engineering Research Board, the Department of Science and Technology, Government of India for lending the support (Grant No. CRG/2021/000126 dated March 11, 2022). SKN, SJ, and PD, PB acknowledge the support of the Honorable Vice-Chancellor of the West Bengal University of Animal and Fishery Sciences, and Jadavpur University, Kolkata, India respectively.

References

[1] Lanza, R., R. Langer, J.P. Vacanti, A. Atala, *Principles of tissue engineering,* Academic press, 2020. Fifth Edition.

[2] Sloan, J.Soft tissue injuries: introduction and basic principles, *Emerg. Med. J. EMJ.* 25 (2008) 33.

[3] Sun, J., X. Ma, F. Li, H. Qi, X. Zhang, Y. Yang, X. Wei, X. Zhao, Debridement and Closure of Soft Tissue Injuries, In: *Tutorials Suturing Tech. Orthop.,* Springer, 2021: pp. 355–375.

[4] Chouhan, D., N. Dey, N. Bhardwaj, B.B. Mandal, Emerging and innovative approaches for wound healing and skin regeneration: Current status and advances, *Biomaterials.* 216 (2019) 119267.

[5] Zarei, F., Soleimaninejad, M. Role of growth factors and biomaterials in wound healing. *Artificial cells, nanomedicine, and biotechnology.* 2018 Oct 31;46(sup1):906-911.

[6] Adair, T.H., J.-P. Montani, Angiogenesis, In: *Colloq. Ser. Integr. Syst. Physiol. from Mol. to Funct.,* 2010: pp. 1–84.

[7] Schirbel, A., S. Kessler, F. Rieder, G. West, N. Rebert, K. Asosingh, C. McDonald, C. Fiocchi, Pro-angiogenic activity of TLRs and NLRs: a novel link between gut microbiota and intestinal angiogenesis, *Gastroenterology.* 144 (2013) 613–623.

[8] Botti, R.H., M. Bossù, N. Zallocco, A. Vestri, A. Polimeni, Effectiveness of plaque indicators and air polishing for the sealing of pits and fissures, *Eur. J. Paediatr. Dent.* 11 (2010) 15.

[9] Ringwood, L., L. Li, The involvement of the interleukin-1 receptor-associated kinases (IRAKs) in cellular signaling networks controlling inflammation, *Cytokine.* 42 (2008) 1–7.

[10] Piraino, F., Selimović Š. A current view of functional biomaterials for wound care, molecular and cellular therapies. *BioMed research international.* 2015 Oct 5;2015.

[11] Sturgeon, R.J. Monosaccharides, In: *Methods Plant Biochem.,* Elsevier, 1990: pp. 1–37.

[12] Avigad, G.A.D. Disaccharides, In: *Methods Plant Biochem.,* Elsevier, 1990: pp. 111–188.

[13] Khowala, S., D. Verma, S.P. Banik, Biomolecules:(Introduction, structure & Function), *Indian Inst. Chem. Biol.* (2008) 3–92.

[14] Gerwig, G.J. Basic Knowledge of Glycobiology, in: *Art Carbohydr. Anal.,* Springer, 2021: pp. 11–50.

[15] Huang, Z., V.B. Kraus, Does lipopolysaccharide-mediated inflammation have a role in OA?, *Nat. Rev. Rheumatol.* 12 (2016) 123–129.

[16] Glasser, W.G. Cellulose and associated heteropolysaccharides, *Glycoscience.* (2008) 1473.

[17] Thangapazham, R.L., Sharad, S., Maheshwari, R.K. Phytochemicals in wound healing. *Advances in wound care.* 2016 May 1;5(5):230-241.

[18] Menor-Salván, C. *Prebiotic chemistry and chemical evolution of nucleic acids,* Springer, 2018.

[19] Ge, Z., H. Gu, Q. Li, C. Fan, Concept and development of framework nucleic acids, *J. Am. Chem. Soc.* 140 (2018) 17808–17819.

[20] Sridharan, K., N.J. Gogtay, Therapeutic nucleic acids: current clinical status, *Br. J. Clin. Pharmacol.* 82 (2016) 659–672.

[21] Harland, A.D., J.C. Navarro, P. Spencer Davies, L.M. Fixter, Lipids of some Caribbean and Red Sea corals: total lipid, wax esters, triglycerides and fatty acids, *Mar. Biol.* 117 (1993) 113–117. https://doi.org/10.1007/BF00346432.

[22] Urban Alandete, L. *Lipid degradation during grain storage: markers, mechanisms and shelf-life extension treatments,* (2019).

[23] Attard, T.M., N. Bukhanko, D. Eriksson, M. Arshadi, P. Geladi, U. Bergsten, V.L. Budarin, J.H. Clark, A.J. Hunt, Supercritical extraction of waxes and lipids from biomass: a valuable first step towards an integrated biorefinery, *J. Clean. Prod.* 177 (2018) 684–698.

[24] Ikada, Y. Challenges in tissue engineering, *J.R. Soc. Interface*. 3 (2006) 589–601.

[25] Santos, M.I., R.L. Reis, Vascularization in bone tissue engineering: physiology, current strategies, major hurdles and future challenges, *Macromol. Biosci.* 10 (2010) 12–27.

[26] Sørensen, O.E., J.B. Cowland, K. Theilgaard-Mönch, L. Liu, T. Ganz, N. Borregaard, Wound Healing and Expression of Antimicrobial Peptides/ Polypeptides in Human Keratinocytes, a Consequence of Common Growth Factors, *J. Immunol.* 170 (2003) 5583 LP – 5589. https://doi.org/10.4049/jimmunol.170.11.5583.

[27] Koria, P. Delivery of growth factors for tissue regeneration and wound healing, *BioDrugs.* 26 (2012) 163–175. https://doi.org/10.2165/11631850-000000000-00000.

[28] Freedman, B.R., D.J. Mooney, Biomaterials to mimic and heal connective tissues, *Adv. Mater.* 31 (2019) 1806695.

[29] Cox, HD., Knussmann G.N., Moore C., Eichner D. Detection of insulin analogues and large peptides> 2 kDa in urine. *Drug Testing and Analysis.* 2022 Jul;14(7): 1264-72.

[30] Teichman, S.L., A. Neale, B. Lawrence, C. Gagnon, J.-P. Castaigne, L.A. Frohman, Prolonged stimulation of growth hormone (GH) and insulin-like growth factor I secretion by CJC-1295, a long-acting analog of GH-releasing hormone, in healthy adults., *J. Clin. Endocrinol. Metab.* 91 (2006) 799–805. https://doi.org/10.1210/jc.2005-1536.

[31] Amini, A., T. Rundlöf, H. Lodén, J.A. Carlsson, M. Lavén, E. Mulugeta, K. Björk, T. Arvidsson, I. Agerkvist, A. Perolari, Identification of Peptides and Proteins in Illegally Distributed Products by MALDI-TOF-MS, in: Mass Spectrom. *Life Sci. Clin.* Lab., IntechOpen, 2021.

[32] Maar, K., R. Hetenyi, S. Maar, G. Faskerti, D. Hanna, B. Lippai, A. Takatsy, I. Bock-Marquette, Utilizing Developmentally Essential Secreted Peptides Such as Thymosin Beta-4 to Remind the Adult Organs of Their Embryonic State—New Directions in Anti-Aging Regenerative Therapies, *Cells.* 10 (2021) 1343.

[33] Tunç, B.S., F. Toprak, S.F. Toprak, S. Sozer, In vitro investigation of growth factors including MGF and IGF-1 in neural stem cell activation, proliferation, and migration, *Brain Res.* 1759 (2021) 147366.

[34] Al-Samerria, S., S. Radovick, The role of insulin-like growth factor-1 (IGF-1) in the control of neuroendocrine regulation of growth, *Cells.* 10 (2021) 2664.

[35] Moreira, F., H. Carmo, P. de Pinho, M. de L. Bastos, Doping detection in animals: A review of analytical methodologies published from 1990 to 2019, *Drug Test. Anal.* 13 (2021) 474–504.

[36] James, O., Friday ET. Phytochemical composition, bioactivity and wound healing potential of Euphorbia heterophylla (Euphorbiaceae) leaf extract. *International Journal on Pharmaceutical and Biomedical Research.* 2010;1(1):54-63.

[37] Peng, Z., R. Xu, Q. You, Role of Traditional Chinese Medicine in Bone Regeneration and Osteoporosis, *Front. Bioeng. Biotechnol.* 10 (2022).

[38] Kosalwatna, S., C. Shaipanich, K. Bhanganada, *The effect of one percent centella asiatica cream on chronic ulcers.*, (1988).

[39] Tejada, S., A. Manayi, M. Daglia, S. F Nabavi, A. Sureda, Z. Hajheydari, O. Gortzi, H. Pazoki-Toroudi, S. M Nabavi, Wound healing effects of curcumin: A short review, *Curr. Pharm. Biotechnol.* 17 (2016) 1002–1007.

[40] Mohanty, C., S.K. Sahoo, Curcumin and its topical formulations for wound healing applications, *Drug Discov. Today.* 22 (2017) 1582–1592.

[41] Chen, C., W. Chiou, J. Zhang, Comparison of the pharmacological effects of Panax ginseng and Panax quinquefolium, *Acta Pharmacol. Sin.* 29 (2008) 1103–1108.

[42] Gil, E.S., B. Panilaitis, E. Bellas, D.L. Kaplan, Functionalized Silk Biomaterials for Wound Healing, *Adv. Healthc. Mater.* 2 (2013) 206–217. https://doi.org/10.1002/ADHM.201200192.

[43] Dan, M.M., P. Sarmah, D.R. Vana, A. Dattatreya, Wound healing: concepts and updates in herbal medicine, *Int J Med Res Heal. Sci.* 7 (2018) 170–181.

[44] Rahimi, M., E.B. Noruzi, E. Sheykhsaran, B. Ebadi, Z. Kariminezhad, M. Molaparast, M.G. Mehrabani, B. Mehramouz, M. Yousefi, R. Ahmadi,

Carbohydrate polymer-based silver nanocomposites: Recent progress in the antimicrobial wound dressings, *Carbohydr. Polym.* 231 (2020) 115696.

[45] Lu, H., X. Li, M. Zhang, C. Xu, W. Li, L. Wan, Antibacterial Cellulose Nanocrystal-Incorporated Hydrogels With Satisfactory Vascularization for Enhancing Skin Regeneration, *Front. Bioeng. Biotechnol.* 10 (2022).

[46] Hao, Y., W. Zhao, L. Zhang, X. Zeng, Z. Sun, D. Zhang, P. Shen, Z. Li, Y. Han, P. Li, Bio-multifunctional alginate/chitosan/fucoidan sponges with enhanced angiogenesis and hair follicle regeneration for promoting full-thickness wound healing, *Mater. Des.* 193 (2020) 108863.

[47] Gao, F., C.X. Yang, W. Mo, Y.W. Liu, Y.Q. He, Hyaluronan oligosaccharides are potential stimulators to angiogenesis via RHAMM mediated signal pathway in wound healing, *Clin. Investig. Med.* (2008) E106–E116. https://doi.org/10.25011/cim.v31i3.3467.

[48] Gao, F., Y. Liu, Y. He, C. Yang, Y. Wang, X. Shi, G. Wei, Hyaluronan oligosaccharides promote excisional wound healing through enhanced angiogenesis, *Matrix Biol.* 29 (2010) 107–116. https://doi.org/10.1016/j.matbio.2009.11.002.

[49] Wang, Y., G. Han, B. Guo, J. Huang, Hyaluronan oligosaccharides promote diabetic wound healing by increasing angiogenesis, *Pharmacol. Reports.* 68 (2016) 1126–1132. https://doi.org/10.1016/j.pharep.2016.07.001.

[50] Li, C., Q. Wang, J. Li, M. Hu, S. Shi, Z. Li, G. Wu, H. Cui, Y. Li, Q. Zhang, X. Yu, L. Lu, Silver nanoparticles/chitosan oligosaccharide/poly(vinyl alcohol) nanofiber promotes wound healing by activating TGFβ1/Smad signaling pathway, *Int. J. Nanomedicine.* 11 (2016) 373–387. https://doi.org/10.2147/IJN.S91975.

[51] Turner, P.R., E. Murray, C.J. McAdam, M.A. McConnell, J.D. Cabral, Peptide chitosan/dextran core/shell vascularized 3D constructs for wound healing, *ACS Appl. Mater. Interfaces.* 12 (2020) 32328–32339.

[52] Padmakumari, R.G., C.D. Sherly, R.M. Ramesan, Therapeutic delivery of nucleic acids for skin wound healing, *Ther. Deliv.* 13 (2022) 339–358.

[53] Wang, Z, Lu H, Tang T, Liu L, Pan B, Chen J, Cheng D, Cai X, Sun Y, Zhu F, Zhu S. Tetrahedral framework nucleic acids promote diabetic wound healing via the Wnt signalling pathway. *Cell Proliferation.* 2022 Nov;55(11):e13316.

[54] Feng, H., Z. Li, W. Xie, Q. Wan, Y. Guo, J. Chen, J. Wang, X. Pei, Delivery of therapeutic miRNAs using nanoscale zeolitic imidazolate framework for accelerating vascularized bone regeneration, *Chem. Eng. J.* 430 (2022) 132867.

[55] Liu, N., X. Zhang, N. Li, M. Zhou, T. Zhang, S. Li, X. Cai, P. Ji, Y. Lin, Tetrahedral framework nucleic acids promote corneal epithelial wound healing in vitro and in vivo, *Small.* 15 (2019) 1901907.

[56] Randeria, P.S., M.A. Seeger, X.-Q. Wang, H. Wilson, D. Shipp, C.A. Mirkin, A.S. Paller, siRNA-based spherical nucleic acids reverse impaired wound healing in diabetic mice by ganglioside GM3 synthase knockdown, *Proc. Natl. Acad. Sci.* 112 (2015) 5573–5578.

[57] Suan Chua, L., N. Abdullah, M.S. Yean Lee, M. Roji Sarmidi, *Review on Labisia pumila (Kacip Fatimah): bioactive phytochemicals and skin collagen synthesis promoting herb,* Elsevier. (2012). https://doi.org/10.1016/j.fitote.2012.04.002.

[58] Auger, FA, Gibot, L, Lacroix, D. The pivotal role of vascularization in tissue engineering. *Annual review of biomedical engineering.* 2013 Jul 11;15:177-200.

[59] Amri, B, Martino E, Vitulo F, Corana F, Ben-Kaâb LB, Rui M, Rossi D, Mori M, Rossi S, Collina S. Marrubium vulgare L. leave extract: Phytochemical composition, antioxidant and wound healing properties. *Molecules.* 2017 Oct 28;22(11):1851.

[60] Amirsadeghi, A., A. Jafari, L.J. Eggermont, S.S. Hashemi, S.A. Bencherif, M. Khorram, Vascularization strategies for skin tissue engineering, *Biomater. Sci.* 8 (2020) 4073–4094. https://doi.org/10.1039/D0BM00266F.

[61] Mahmoud, M.F., D.M. Monti, S. Vitale, S. Colanero, M. Placidi, G. Di Emidio, C. Tatone, F. Amicarelli, A. Maria D'alessandro, Phytochemistry and Biological Activity of Medicinal Plants in Wound Healing: An Overview of Current Research, *Mdpi.Com.* 27 (2022) 27. https://doi.org/10.3390/molecules27113566.

[62] Chen, S. Natural products triggering biological targets-a review of the anti-inflammatory phytochemicals targeting the arachidonic acid pathway in allergy asthma and rheumatoid arthritis. C*urrent drug targets.* 2011 Mar 1;12(3):288-301.

[63] Burnouf, T., H. Goubran, K.-L. Ou, H.A. Goubran, T.-M. Chen, M. El-Ekiaby, M. *Radosevic, Blood-derived biomaterials and platelet growth factors in regenerative medicine,* Elsevier. (2013). https://doi.org/10.1016/j.blre.2013.02.001.

[64] Pei, Y., L. Zhang, X. Mao, Z. Liu, W. Cui, X. Sun, Y. Zhang, Biomaterial Scaffolds for Improving Vascularization During Skin Flap Regeneration, Chinese *J. Plast. Reconstr. Surg.* 2 (2020) 109–119. https://doi.org/10.1016/S2096-6911(21)00021-2.

[65] Nurkesh, A, Jaguparov, A, Jimi, S, Saparov, A. Recent advances in the controlled release of growth factors and cytokines for improving cutaneous wound healing. *Frontiers in Cell and Developmental Biology.* 2020 Jul 14;8:638.

Chapter 2

The Role of Oxygenation in Tissue Engineering

Aysegul Gencer*, MD
Istanbul Bakirkoy Dr. Sadi Konuk Training and Research Hospital,
Department of Chest Diseases, Istanbul, Turkey

Abstract

The delivery of oxygen to the human body, which is an essential requirement for the survival of cells, is carried out by the respiratory system. The alveolar surfaces constitute the gas diffusion area. Oxygenation of blood is carried out according to simple diffusion rules through the blood-air barrier. It is presented to the tissues by the circulatory system, the first developing system in the embryonic period.

There must be no ventilation/perfusion disorder at the stage of providing adequate oxygen to the tissues. Diseases that disrupt this balance, such as chronic obstructive pulmonary disease, asthma, pulmonary embolism, and pulmonary edema, cause hypoxemia in tissue. A decrease in tissue oxygen, an essential factor in tissue healing and development, will impair or even stop tissue repair.

In tissue engineering, where new steps are taken in producing biomaterials for repairing and regenerating damaged tissues and failed organs, all risk factors that impair oxygenation and perfusion should be evaluated since tissue repair is essential in increasing the survival of the biomaterial.

Keywords: endothelial dysfunction, tissue engineering, oxygen delivery, tissue healing, hypoxemia

---

* Corresponding Author's Email: aysegulbozkurtgencer@gmail.com.

In: Vascularization and Its Role in Medicine and Tissue Engineering
Editors: Emre Bulbul and Murat Oguz Ozilhan
ISBN: 979-8-89113-041-8

Introduction

Most of the energy required for the human body's survival is realized through chemical reactions in the cells using oxygen. The basic system that provides the oxygen required for this process is the respiratory system. The respiratory tract is divided into the upper and lower respiratory tract. The upper respiratory tract consists of the nasal cavity, paranasal sinuses, pharynx, and larynx; the lower respiratory tract consists of the trachea, bronchi, lobular and terminal bronchioles, respiratory bronchioles and terminates in alveoli [1]. The function of the upper respiratory tract is to filter, warm, and humidify the inhaled air. The lower respiratory tract is where gas exchange occurs [2]. The alveoli, the endpoints of the bronchioles, create an area of approximately 150m2 for gas diffusion due to their shape [3, 4]. One of the main functions of the respiratory system is to transmit inhaled air to the alveoli, thus taking in oxygen and removing carbon dioxide.

Venous blood, pumped by the right ventricle, reaches the blood-air barrier after extending from the main pulmonary arteries to the alveolar capillaries. The pulmonary artery and veins that carry deoxygenated blood and oxygenated blood to the heart, respectively, constitute the pulmonary vascular structure of the lungs [5]. Oxygenated blood in the pulmonary capillaries reaches the left atrium with the pulmonary veins and is pumped throughout the body. With each breath, 500 ml of air is taken, 250 ml of CO_2 per minute passes into the alveoli, and 300 ml of oxygen into the capillaries.

Gas exchange is provided in the septum, the blood-air barrier between the alveoli and the pulmonary capillaries [6]. The blood-air barrier is a relatively simple structure consisting of 3 layers: Alveolar epithelium, extracellular matrix, and capillary endothelium. A thin aqueous layer on the epithelial surface reduces the surface tension. Type 4 collagen in the extracellular matrix provides the necessary strength for the barrier [7].

The principle of gas transition with simple diffusion from high to low pressure is valid for gas diffusion through this blood-air barrier. The richer the inspired air is from oxygen, the more oxygen passes through the blood-air barrier and the greater oxygenation [8, 9]. According to Fick's law of diffusion, diffusion of a gas across the alveolar membrane increases with the following:

- Increased membrane surface area
- The increased alveolar pressure difference
- Increased gas solubility

- Decreased membrane thickness

Oxygen delivery to the tissue is ensured with adequate ventilation and perfusion. Adequate ventilation and perfusion of the alveoli are required for effective gas exchange [10]. Ventilation is the airflow from the outside into the alveoli, while perfusion is blood flow into the capillary.

Ventilation is 50% greater at the base of the lung than at the apex. The negative pressure of physiological fluid in the pleural space is less in the basal. This results in a further increase in alveolar volume in the basal inspiration. On the other hand, perfusion is more significant in the basal, as it depends entirely on gravity. The increase in basal perfusion is more significant than ventilation [11]. When the ventilation/perfusion ratio increases, the arterial blood's partial oxygen, and carbon dioxide pressure increase and decrease, respectively. At a low ventilation/perfusion ratio, it will act in the opposite direction [12]. Changes in ventilation to perfusion ratio can affect gas exchange and ultimately cause hypoxemia [13].

Hypoxemia

Hypoxemia is defined as a decrease in oxygen carried in the arterial blood. There are four mechanisms involved in the development of hypoxemia [14]:

- Ventilation/perfusion defect: it is the most common cause of hypoxemia [15]
- A gas exchange defect in the alveolo-capillary membrane causes diffusion disorder.
- Alveolar hypoventilation: The characteristic of hyperventilation is detecting a high partial carbon dioxide pressure [16].
- Increased shunt: Shunt is the passage of blood from the right heart to the left without any gas exchange. It is an excessive ventilation-perfusion (V/Q) mismatch without ventilation. A shunt can be considered in the presence of no response to oxygen therapy [17].

It is known that conditions that disrupt the ventilation/perfusion balance in the lungs, such as smoking for a long time, cause hypoxia and delay tissue healing. Conditions causing ventilation/perfusion disturbance:

- Ventilation/perfusion defect is expected in cardiac conditions such as pulmonary arterio-venous malformations and congenital heart diseases.
- In chronic obstructive pulmonary disease, the most important causes of hypoxemia are ventilation-perfusion defect due to progressive airway stenosis and diffusion disorder secondary to emphysematous destruction of the pulmonary capillary bed [18].
- Asthma-related bronchoconstriction reduces the ventilation/perfusion rate. Supplemental oxygen therapy is required in addition to bronchodilator treatments to bring the balance back to normal limits.
- Pulmonary embolism is one of the most important causes of ventilation/perfusion disorder. It causes non-perfusable alveoli. This will result in hypoxemia [19].
- Hypoxemia in pulmonary fibrosis is due to ventilation/perfusion disorder, increased shunt, and limited diffusion [20].
- The walls of the alveoli in the lung become thicker due to fluid filling on the surfaces, and gas exchange is impaired in pulmonary edema. Edema causes hypoxemia by preventing the ventilated air from reaching the capillaries, preventing ventilation, and impairing perfusion.

These causes due to ventilation/perfusion disorder or diffusion abnormality can be regressed with oxygen support therapy [21].

Hypoxia-Related Respiratory Diseases Caused by Ventilation/Perfusion Defects

Chronic Obstructive Pulmonary Disease

Chronic obstructive pulmonary disease (COPD) progresses with chronic cough, chronic sputum production, and dyspnea in individuals with risk factors such as smoking, biomass exposure, and occupational exposure [22].

Long-term smoking causes respiratory tract inflammation. This inflammation will predispose to chronic obstructive pulmonary disease. It causes emphysema by causing parenchymal tissue destruction and fibrosis in small airways due to deterioration in repair and defence mechanisms. These changes will cause progressive airway restriction and air trapping in the long term [23].

In addition to this pathogenesis secondary to immune response, other mechanisms are still waiting to be clarified in the pathogenesis of COPD. Pathology and pathophysiology can be summarized as follows:

- Oxidative stress: It is accepted as one of the important predisposing factors in pathogenesis. Cigarette smoking has a long-term effect on reducing antioxidant production. Reactive oxygen species produced in these patients increase with smoking and the frequency of exacerbations [24].
- Protease-antiprotease balance: An increase in protease levels produced by inflammatory and epithelial cells was detected due to the inflammatory response. These proteases, which will destroy the main components of the lung parenchyma, namely elastin, will play a role in the development of emphysema [25].
- Inflammatory cells and mediators: Both the number of macrophages and the number of neutrophils and lymphocytes increase in lung tissue and thickened airways in COPD. Epithelial cells also secrete many inflammatory mediators along with all these inflammatory cells [26]. As a result, structural changes are induced in the lung with the increase of the inflammatory process [27].
- Fibrosis: The remodelling process occurs due to lung tissue damage caused by recurrent inflammation, and muscle and fibrous tissue production increases. It is thought that this fibrosis process contributes to the narrowing of the small airway and the development of emphysema [28].
- Airway limitation and air trapping: Thickened airway causes airway limitation. Hyperinflation occurs as a result of progressive airway limitation. At this point, the patient feels dyspnea [29].
- Gas diffusion disorder: Tissue damage due to emphysema causes a decrease in gas transfer. Decreased ventilation in progressive disease will increase dead air space. The increased respiratory effort with decreased ventilation will cause carbon dioxide retention and impaired ventilation/perfusion ratio [30].

Asthma Causing Bronchoconstriction

Carbon dioxide retention increases, and respiratory alkalosis occurs with the development of bronchoconstriction and fatigue in the respiratory muscles in asthma. V/Q mismatch is the primary mechanism of gas exchange abnormality in asthma [31]. There can be remodelling of pulmonary vascular structures and airway remodelling in long-standing, untreated, or inadequately treated asthma. This leads to permanent perfusion abnormalities [32]. Bronchoconstriction, diffuse peripheral airway edema, and mucus obstruction are also thought to be responsible for ventilation/perfusion abnormalities in acute asthma [33].

Pulmonary Embolism

Acute pulmonary embolism disrupts the oxygen-carbon dioxide gas diffusion in the blood-air barrier. It causes a decrease in arterial partial pressure of oxygen, namely hypoxemia. Since perfusion of pulmonary arteries occluded by embolism will be impaired, ventilation/perfusion defect occurs in these regions. Total dead space increases as ventilation continues, while perfusion decreases in patients with acute pulmonary embolism. Since carbon dioxide cannot be removed in the increasing dead space, the clinical manifestation progresses to hypercapnia [34].

Pulmonary Fibrosis

The most common gas diffusion problem in pulmonary fibrosis is hypoxemia without hypercapnia [35]. Although the cause of hypoxemia is the coexistence of V/Q mismatch, shunt, and diffusion restriction, V/Q mismatch is the most common cause [36].

Pulmonary Edema

Fluid accumulating in the alveoli in pulmonary edema is one of the most important causes of diffusion disorder. The thickness of the alveolar wall increases with the increased amount of fluid. The gas exchange surface area in the alveoli is reduced. Edema prevents ventilated air from reaching the capillaries. As a result, ventilation/perfusion defect occurs. There are many causes of pulmonary edema. Heart failure, nephrotic syndrome, kidney failure, hepatic failure, ARDS, sepsis, and many similar conditions can cause this clinical picture [37].

The Relationship between Tissue Healing and Hypoxemia

Effective wound healing includes the following events: 1- hemostasis, 2- inflammation, 3- mesenchymal cell differentiation, proliferation, and migration to the wound site, 4- angiogenesis, 5- epithelialization, and 6- remodelling [38, 39].

Many factors affect tissue healing. Oxygenation is one of the local factors. It is essential for cell metabolism, especially energy production. It plays a role in almost all wound healing steps. It reduces the risk of infection, induces angiogenesis, increases keratinocyte differentiation, migration, and epithelialization promotes fibroblast proliferation and collagen synthesis [40, 41].

As a result, impaired oxygenation of tissues causes impaired tissue repair. It depends on three essential conditions to ensure tissue oxygenation: 1- oxygenation of arterial blood, 2- delivery of oxygen to the tissue, and 3- oxygen use by tissue. Arterial partial oxygen pressure is the most reliable parameter for evaluating tissue oxygenation [42]. Decreased partial oxygen pressure in arterial blood is defined as hypoxemia.

Good perfusion and oxygenation are essential in healthy tissue healing and repair. It is known that a moist and oxygenated wound-healing environment increases the epithelialization rate of the wound up to 3 times [43]. Epidermal cells grow at an oxygenation concentration ranging from 20-50% [44].

Good oxygenation is required to release collagen, one of the main components of wound healing, and for the hydroxylation of proline and lysine for its association with fibroblasts. Wound healing is delayed in hypoxemia.

Collagen synthesis in tissue healing is closely related to the oxygen concentration in the tissue. Potential mechanisms are thought to be in the details of collagen biosynthesis and post-translational modification. Four oxygen-related enzymes modify collagen production: prolyl 4-hydroxylase, prolyl 3-hydroxylase, lysyl hydroxylase, and lysyl oxidase [45]. Proline and lysine hydroxylase is involved in collagen production, cross-linking, and strengthening of scar tissue, and the oxygen concentration required for enzyme activity varies between 20-100mm Hg [46]. The hydroxylation of proline by 4-prolyl hydroxylase is correlated with collagen synthesis. Hydroxylation is delayed when the concentration of oxygen decreases and the pro-alpha chain of collagen is synthesized as a non-functional protein [47]. Low hydroxylated collagen accumulated in hypoxic patients has limited contribution to tissue strength. In addition, angiogenesis of tissue correlates with the partial pressure of oxygen in the blood. Many steps in wound healing and synthesis, deposition, and cross-linking of collagen are closely related to oxygenation and perfusion.

It has been shown that increasing the oxygen concentration in the inhaled air to 80% with oxygen support therapy supports tissue repair and reduces the infection rate by half compared to %30 oxygen concentration [48]. Higher-pressure hyperbaric oxygen therapy enhances epidermopoiesis through fibroblast proliferation and differentiation of keratinocytes [49].

Supplemental oxygen therapy should be given after surgeries to improve oxygenation and perfusion of traumatized tissues. In hyperbaric oxygen therapy, pure oxygen increases the diffusion distance of oxygen in the tissue by 3 to 4 times [50]. Although hyperbaric oxygen therapy has little effect on the healing of normally uncomplicated wounds, it is thought to be effective in complicated ischemic wounds.

Anemia also has a negative effect on tissue healing. Since the oxygen available to the wound is low, cardiac output increases to enhance the perfusion. The balance is tried to be maintained by rapid perfusion as arterial partial oxygen decreases. However, if this problem cannot be resolved with perfusion, there will be problems in tissue healing. A hemoglobin value of more than ten g/dL is recommended for tissue healing. This is important to increase the perfusion of the tissue, significantly increasing the oxygen concentration [51].

The Relationship between Tissue Healing and Perfusion

Perfusion of tissues is highly dependent on external factors. Cold, heat, pain, fear, and other medical reasons, mainly smoking, affect perfusion. Perfusion disorders due to these factors are common, especially during and after surgery [52].

Tobacco smoke contains more than 4000 toxins or carcinogenic chemicals. It is associated with cardiovascular and lung diseases, immune system diseases, cancer, and impaired wound healing [53]. Smoking increases the risk of tissue necrosis, especially after surgery, and the risk of infection [54]. Nicotine is absorbed by smoking. Catecholamine release begins and causes vasoconstriction, resulting in a 42% decrease in perfusion. Besides, the oxygen concentration in the blood will also decrease due to the CO in tobacco smoke. Even with one cigarette, a 30% reduction in tissue perfusion for about one minute has been shown [55]. Collagen production is also less in these areas where perfusion is reduced in smokers [56].

Based on clinical observations, it is known that wounds in well-perfused tissues heal faster than in non-perfused tissues. Continuous oxygen support accelerates wound healing in well-perfused tissues and provides resistance to infection. Good vascularization and tissue oxygenation due to tissue perfusion accelerate the regression of tissue damage.

Angiogenesis

Angiogenesis, defined as the formation of blood vessel structures, consists of 3 stages. These stages are vasculogenesis, angiogenesis, and arteriogenesis. In vasculogenesis, primaries of blood vessels are formed by the differentiation of mesodermal progenitor cells and angioblasts [57]. In angiogenesis, capillaries extending from existing vascular structures develop. Mesodermal progenitor cells do not need to be involved. Arteriovenous, known as collateral development, occurs as an adaptive response to transient situations [58]. The data presented in terms of the formation steps of angiogenesis have been instructive for tissue engineering.

Angioblasts are precursor cells of vascular structures. In angiogenesis, which is the formation of vascular structures, arterial, capillary and venous networks are formed from large vascular structures to small ones [59]. Angiogenesis is initiated or stopped by several stimulating and inhibitory factors. The presence of tissue ischemia, trauma, hypoxia, or tumour triggers angiogenesis, and the expression of proangiogenic growth factors increases with their activated receptors. Vascular permeability increases in response to vascular endothelial growth factors (VEGF). Thus, plasma proteins are extravasated, and primitive endothelial cell migration is achieved [60, 61]. During this process, while angiopoietin -1 inhibits vascular permeability, angiopoietin-2 increases permeability by showing an antagonistic effect. After that, matrix metalloproteinase degrades matrix components to increase angiogenesis. Migrating endothelial cells aggregate to form a cord. Integrin promotes the migration and adhesion of endothelial cells. Vascular endothelial-cadherin both promotes adhesion and increases survival [62]. When the cord and the vessel are formed, they are supported by smooth muscle cells and pericytes. Angiopoietin -1, platelet-derived growth factor (PDGF)-B, and PDGF receptor have a role in their maturation. This process, which is completed by the expansion of the lumen, is called arteriogenesis [63].

Hypoxia and Angiogenesis

Angiogenesis is a series of processes that can develop due to many triggers and occur with the activation of many proangiogenic factors. In particular, any condition that can cause hypoxia triggers angiogenesis [63]. Cellular stress secondary to hypoxia provides activation of the genetic cascade. Hypoxia-inducible factor (HIF)-1 is a hypoxia-induced angiogenetic transcription factor [64, 65].

Oxygen Delivery

Oxygen is essential for tissue development, healing, and homeostasis. Therefore, the circulatory system is the first developed system during the embryonic period. Oxygen homeostasis management is essential to provide the tissues with sufficient oxygen and to establish a balance with toxic oxidants [66]. In the case of hypoxia, where the oxygen concentration is reduced, several genes will activate for angiogenesis, cell survival, proliferation, and regulation of glucose and iron metabolism.

Hypoxia-Inducible Factor-1

In tissues where hypoxia develops, a series of gene activations occur for the survival of cells. HIF-1 is the primary transcriptional mediator in cell response to hypoxia. HIF-1 regulates gene expressions related to oxygen transport, glucose metabolism, and angiogenesis. This transcription factor regulates erythropoietin (EPO) expression at low oxygen levels. HIF-1 consists of two subunits: HIF-1 *α and HIF-1 β. HIF-1 β is a more structural subunit.*

On the other hand, HIF-1 α contains a domain for DNA binding in response to hypoxia. There are three known isoforms of HIF-α. HIF-2α and

HIF-3α together with the isoform HIF-1α. HIF-2α is found constitutively in endothelium, cartilage, and lung. HIF-3α, also called inhibitory Per-ARNT-Sim, *is a negative regulator that inactivates the binding site of DNA [67].*

Vasculogenesis, Angiogenesis, and Hypoxic Conditions

Oxygen concentration plays an essential role in the vasculogenesis of the embryo. Before the development of the circulatory system, which is the first system that develops during the embryonic process, the oxygen concentration is at low levels. Since an increase in oxygen level is required for development, the formation of primitive vascular structures from angioblasts begins.

It has been shown that hypoxia and the expression of HIF-1 contribute to angiogenesis by activating angiogenic genes and receptors (VEGF, placental growth factor, PDGFB, Angiopoietin-1, and Angiopoietin-2). It regulates proangiogenic chemokines (stromal cell-derived factor 1α, sphingosine-1-phosphate, and receptors CXCR4, C-X-C chemokine receptor type 4, and sphingosine-1-phosphate receptors). In brief, HIF-1 plays a crucial role in the process of angiogenesis and is involved in every step of angiogenesis. VEGF are primary factors for the regulation of angiogenesis. HIF-1 is the main stimulator of VEGF [68].

HIF-1 accumulates in the presence of hypoxia in the tissue, and HIF-1 upregulates VEGF, the major proangiogenic factor. If the oxygen balance is disturbed, it will bind to VEGF receptors and trigger vascular development. However, if tissue perfusion is adequate, the tissue will be normoxic, and it can be assumed that the cascade will cease. When hypoxia cannot be relieved with increased perfusion, the extracellular matrix will be degraded by metalloproteinases, and endothelial cell migration and formation of vascular tubular structures will be allowed. Expression of metalloproteinase two is also induced by HIF-1 [69]. In the third step, endothelial cell proliferation and adhesion occur. This is induced by integrin αβ. HIF-1 controls the endothelial cell behaviour at this stage [70]. In the last step, vascular maturation, the basal membrane is formed by collecting pericytes and smooth muscle cells. Thus the angiogenesis process is completed.

Oxygen Delivery in Tissue Engineering

Tissue engineering aims to develop replacement tissue grafts and new biomaterials for clinical use in repairing and regenerating damaged tissues and failed organs. Although there have been significant developments in this field in recent years, there are still severe difficulties. The circulatory system plays a role in providing oxygen for the survival of tissues in physiological conditions. Thus, angiogenesis is essential for the survival of these new biomaterials in damaged tissue [71]. In addition, there are limitations to the vascularization of in vitro or in vivo tissues at the point where tissue engineering has reached. In particular, oxygen diffusion problems are one of these limitations. From this point of view, many studies have been carried out on vascularization in tissue engineering.

In vitro vascularization of tissues is currently the main focus of tissue engineering. Perfusion and oxygen transport have direct effects on cell viability and differentiation. Oxygen and nutrient diffusion are necessary for the metabolic needs of the tissue. Combined approaches with vascularization, such as local oxygen support, should be considered in tissue engineering. More functional vascular structures can be created by reducing capillary spaces and increasing the oxygen rate after implicating vascular cells into engineered tissue [72].

A study using oxygen-producing bioengineered materials aimed to show that tissue engineering can increase tissue survival. It has been mentioned that it can help prevent problems in oxygen diffusion, especially in large tissue implants [73].

Although the idea for success in tissue engineering is to keep the oxygen support at the highest level, studies have shown that moderate oxygenation of tissue in vitro conditions gives a better response than high oxygen levels. Hyperoxia can cause cell damage due to the production of reactive oxygen species. It may also slow down cell growth and proliferation, resulting in apoptosis. While angiogenesis is supported by preventing hypoxia in tissue engineering, the optimal value should be found in oxygenation, and high levels should be avoided [74].

Smoking and Hypoxic Lung Diseases in Tissue Engineering

It has been shown that smokers' endothelial progenitor, hematopoietic stem, and progenitor cell functions are impaired in vitro ischemia models created to evaluate endothelial cell survival and vascular morphogenesis show that perfusion of ischemic tissues can be improved in non-smokers. At the same time, this therapeutic effect is lost in smokers. It has been shown that endothelial cell survival and proliferation are decreased due to smoking in vitro vasculogenesis. In conclusion, smokers are at risk for both in vivo therapeutic activity and in vitro vasculogenic activity [75]. Smoking prevents the increase of perfusion in ischemic tissue and decreases vasculogenic activity due to the increased level of Activin A, which is an angiostatic factor. For these reasons, serious difficulties may be experienced in the survival of tissue-engineered biomaterials in a patient with a history of excessive smoking. In these patients, oxygen-generating biomaterials should be considered in addition to treatment options ranging from supplemental oxygen therapy to hyperbaric oxygen therapy.

In diseases such as chronic obstructive pulmonary disease, which is characterized by tissue destruction in the lung structure, impaired ventilation/perfusion balance, and hypoxemia, the amount of oxygen reaching the tissue will be low despite the vascularization in tissues due to triggered hypoxemia and the repair of the tissue will slow down or even stop Asthma, pulmonary embolism, and many medical conditions leading to pulmonary edema will also have a pathophysiology similar to ventilation/perfusion dysfunction. Smoking status and comorbidities that may cause ventilation/perfusion disorders will significantly reduce tissue repair success in patients planning for tissue engineering.

Self-Oxygenation of Tissue-Engineered Living Implants

In tissue engineering, tissue viability is high in small implants, whereas failure is more common in large implants. While small implants can provide oxygen and nutrient diffusion from the host, large implants remain anoxic, and thus failure is inevitable [76]. While hypoxia is a promoter of angiogenesis, anoxia inhibits these regenerative processes and causes cell death [77].

Including an oxygen delivery system in the implants will break the anoxia, create a state of hypoxia, and trigger vascularization. However, this requires a prolonged and controlled release of oxygen. Various oxygen release and generation strategies, such as hemoglobin and myoglobin substitutes, polymer-based oxygen carriers, perfluorocarbons, and solid peroxides, have been developed in this context [78].

Conclusion

Since tissue repair is essential in increasing the survival of the biomaterial in tissue engineering, where new steps are taken in the production of biomaterials in the repair and regeneration of damaged tissues and failed organs, all factors and diseases that impair oxygenation and perfusion will lead the tissue to failure. All conditions that may cause hypoxemia and prevent angiogenesis should be investigated in patients. Oxygen support therapy and hyperbaric oxygen therapy can increase the success rate. The use of oxygen-producing tissue-engineered biomaterials, believed to be beneficial in preventing problems of oxygen diffusion in large tissue implants, should be evaluated in these patients.

References

[1] Moore K L, Dalley A F, Agur A M. *Clinically oriented anatomy.* Lippincott Williams & Wilkins; 2013 Feb 13.

[2] Burri, Peter H. "Structural aspects of postnatal lung development–alveolar formation and growth." *Neonatology* 89.4 (2006): 313-322.

[3] Tyler, Walter S. "Comparative subgross anatomy of lungs: Pleural, interlobular septa, and distal airways." *American Review of Respiratory Disease* 128.2P2 (1983): 32-S36.

[4] Fréchette, Éric, Jean Deslauriers. "Surgical anatomy of the bronchial tree and pulmonary artery." *Seminars in thoracic and cardiovascular surgery.* Vol. 18. No. 2. WB Saunders, 2006.

[5] Smith, Una, J. W. Ryan. "Substructural features of pulmonary endothelial caveolae." *Tissue and Cell* 4.1 (1972): 49-54.

[6] Yoneda, Kokichi. "Regional differences in the intercellular junctions of the alveolar-capillary membrane in the human lung." *American Review of Respiratory Disease* 126.5 (1982): 893-897.

[7] Timpl R, Wiedemann H, van Delden V, Furthmayr H, Kühn K. A network model for the organization of type IV collagen molecules in basement membranes. *Eur. J. Biochem.* 120: 203– 211, 1981.

[8] Meyrick, Barbara, Lynne Reid. "Ultrastructural findings in lung biopsy material from children with congenital heart defects." *The American Journal of Pathology* 101.3 (1980): 527.

[9] Lauweryns, J. M. "The blood and lymphatic microcirculation of the lung." *Pahol. Ann.* 6 (1971): 365-415

[10] Powers K A, Dhamoon A S. *Physiology, Pulmonary Ventilation, and Perfusion.* [2022 Jan 28]. StatPearls Publishing; 2022 Jan

[11] Wagner P.D, Laravuso R.B, Uhl R.R, West J.B. Continuous distributions of ventilation-perfusion ratios in normal subjects breathing air and 100 percent O2. *J. Clin. Invest.* 1974 Jul;54(1):54-68

[12] Petersson J, Glenny RW. Gas exchange and ventilation-perfusion relationships in the lung. *Eur. Respir. J.* 2014 Oct;44(4):1023-41.

[13] Wagner P.D, Laravuso R.B, Uhl R.R, West J.B. Continuous distributions of ventilation-perfusion ratios in normal subjects breathing air and 100 percent O2. *J. Clin. Invest.* 1974 Jul;54(1):54-68.

[14] Roussos C., A. Koutsoukou Respiratory failure. *Eur. Respir. J.,* 22 (2003), pp. 3s-14s, 10.1183/09031936.03.00038503.

[15] Belda J F, Soro M, Ferrando C. Pathophysiology of respiratory failure. *Trends Anaesth. Crit. Care.* 2013;3:265–9.

[16] Williams A J. ABC of oxygen: Assessing and interpreting arterial blood gases and acid-base balance. *BMJ.* 1998;317:1213–6.

[17] Patel A J, Lazdunski M, Honoré E. Kv2.1/Kv9.3, a novel ATP-dependent delayed-rectifier K+ channel in oxygen-sensitive pulmonary artery myocytes. *EMBO J.* 1997;16:6615–6625.

[18] Gibson G J. *Clinical Tests of Respiratory Function.* 3rd ed. London: Hodder Arnold; 2009.

[19] Huet Y, Lemaire F, Brun-Buisson C, Knaus WA, Teisseire B, Payen D, Mathieu D. Hypoxemia in acute pulmonary embolism. *Chest.* 1985 Dec;88(6):829-36.

[20] Javaheri S, Sicilian L. Lung function, breathing pattern, and gas exchange in interstitial lung disease. *Thorax.* 1992;47:93–97.

[21] Frizzelli, R., Lettieri, C., Caiola, S., Maulucci, L., Pinzi, C., Agostini, F., Frizzelli, A. (2022). Unexplained hypoxemia in COPD with cardiac shunt. *Respiratory Medicine Case Reports,* 37, 101661.

[22] Stafinski, T., Nagase, F. I., Avdagovska, M., Stickland, M. K., Menon, D. (2022). Effectiveness of home-based pulmonary rehabilitation programs for patients with chronic obstructive pulmonary disease (COPD): systematic review. *BMC Health Services Research*, 22(1), 1-14.

[23] Hogg J C, Timens W. The pathology of chronic obstructive pulmonary disease. *Annu. Rev. Pathol.* 2009;4:435-59. doi: 10.1146/annurev.pathol.4.110807.092145. PMID: 18954287.

[24] Kirkham P A, Barnes P J. Oxidative stress in COPD. *Chest.* 2013 Jul;144(1):266-273. DOI: 10.1378/chest.12-2664. PMID: 23880677.

[25] Johnson S R. Untangling the protease web in COPD: metalloproteinases in the silent zone. *Thorax.* 2016 Feb;71(2):105-6. doi: 10.1136/thoraxjnl-2015-208204. PMID: 26769014.

[26] Barnes P J. Inflammatory mechanisms in patients with chronic obstructive pulmonary disease. *J. Allergy Clin. Immunol.* 2016 Jul;138(1):16-27. doi: 10.1016/j.jaci.2016.05.011. Epub 2016 May 27. PMID: 27373322.

[27] Barnes P J. Cellular and molecular mechanisms of chronic obstructive pulmonary disease. *Clin. Chest Med.* 2014 Mar;35(1):71-86. doi: 10.1016/j.ccm.2013.10.004. Epub 2013 Dec 12. PMID: 24507838.

[28] Rennard S I, Wachenfeldt K V. Rationale and emerging approaches for targeting lung repair and regeneration in the treatment of chronic obstructive pulmonary disease. *Proc. Am. Thorac. Soc.* 2011 Aug;8(4):368-75. doi: 10.1513/pats.201102-019RM. PMID: 21816994

[29] Ofir D, Laveneziana P, Webb K A, Lam Y M, O'Donnell D E. Mechanisms of dyspnea during cycle exercise in symptomatic patients with GOLD stage I chronic obstructive pulmonary disease. *Am. J. Respir. Crit. Care Med.* 2008 Mar 15;177(6): 622-9. Doi: 10.1164/rccm.200707-1064OC. Epub 2007 Nov 15. PMID: 18006885

[30] Rodríguez-Roisin R, Drakulovic M, Rodríguez D A, Roca J, Barberà J A, Wagner PD. Ventilation-perfusion imbalance and chronic obstructive pulmonary disease staging severity. *J. Appl. Physiol.* (1985). 2009 Jun;106(6):1902-8. doi: 10.1152/japplphysiol.00085.2009. Epub 2009 Apr 16. PMID: 19372303.

[31] Wagner P D, Dantzker D R, Iacovoni V E, Tomlin WC, West JB. Ventilation-perfusion inequality in asymptomatic asthma. *Am. Rev. Respir. Dis.* 1978;118:511–24.

[32] Harris R S, Winkler T, Tgavalekos N, Musch G, Melo M F, Schroeder T, Chang Y, Venegas JG. Regional pulmonary perfusion, inflation, and ventilation defects in bronchoconstricted patients with asthma. *Am. J. Respir. Crit. Care Med.* 2006 Aug 1;174(3):245-53. Doi: 10.1164/rccm.200510-1634OC. Epub 2006 May 11. PMID: 16690973; PMCID: PMC2648114.

[33] Parameswaran K, Knight A C, Keaney N P, Williams E D, Taylor I K. Ventilation and perfusion lung scintigraphy of allergen-induced airway responses in atopic asthmatic subjects. *Can. Respir. J.* 2007 Jul-Aug;14(5):285-91. Doi: 10.1155/2007/474202. PMID: 17703244; PMCID: PMC2676395.

[34] Goldhaber, S. Z., Elliott, C. G. (2003). Acute pulmonary embolism: part I: epidemiology, pathophysiology, and diagnosis. *Circulation*, *108*(22), 2726-2729.

[35] Agustí A G, Barberà J A. Contribution of multiple inert gas elimination technique to pulmonary medicine 2.Chronic pulmonary diseases: Chronic obstructive pulmonary disease and idiopathic pulmonary fibrosis. *Thorax.* 1994;49:924–32.

[36] Agustí A G, Roca J, Gea J, Wagner P D, Xaubet A, Rodriguez-Roisin R. Mechanisms of gas-exchange impairment in idiopathic pulmonary fibrosis. *Am. Rev. Respir. Dis.* 1991;143:219–25.

[37] Powers K A, Dhamoon A S. *Physiology, Pulmonary Ventilation, and Perfusion.* [Updated 2022 Jan 28]. StatPearls Publishing; 2022 Jan.

[38] Gosain A, DiPietro LA. (2004). Aging and wound healing. *World J. Surg.* 28:321-326.

[39] Mathieu D, Linke J-C, Wattel F. (2006). Non-healing wounds. In: *Handbook on hyperbaric medicine*, Mathieu DE, editor. Netherlands: Springer, pp. 401-427.

[40] Bishop A. (2008). Role of oxygen in wound healing. *J. Wound Care* 17:399-402.

[41] Rodriguez P G, Felix F N, Woodley D T, Shim E K. (2008). The role of oxygen in wound healing: a review of the literature. *Dermatol Surg* 34:1159-1169.

[42] F Gottrup (1994) Physiology and measurement of tissue perfusion *Ann. Chir. Gynecol.* 83 183–1891.

[43] Wiseman, D. M. (1992). Wound dressings: design and use. *Wound healing: biochemical and clinical aspects*, 562-580.

[44] Horikoshi, T., Balin, A. K., Carter, D. M. (1986). Effect of oxygen on the growth of human epidermal keratinocytes. *Journal of investigative dermatology*, 86(4), 424-427.

[45] Jonsson K E, Jensen J A, Goodson 3rd W H, Scheuenstuhl H E, West J U, Hopf H W, Hunt T K. Tissue oxygenation, anemia, and perfusion in relation to wound healing in surgical patients. *Annals of surgery*. 1991 Nov;214(5):605.

[46] Gottrup, F. Oxygen in Wound Healing and Infection. *World J. Surg*. 28, 312–315 (2004). https://doi.org/10.1007/s00268-003-7398-5.

[47] Prockop DJ, Kivirikko KI, Tuderman L, Guzman NA. The bio- synthesis of collagen and its disorders,Part I. *N. Engl. J. Med.* 1979; 301(1):13-23.

[48] Greif R, Akça O, Horn E P, Kurz A, Sessler DI. Supplemental perioperative oxygen to reduce the incidence of surgical-wound infection. *New England Journal of Medicine*. 2000 Jan 20;342(3):161-7.

[49] Dan Dimitrijevich S, Paranjape S, Wilson J R, Gracy R W, Mills J G. Effect of hyperbaric oxygen on human skin cells in culture and in human dermal and skin equivalents. *Wound Repair and Regeneration*. 1999 Jan;7(1):53-64.

[50] Sheffield P J. Measuring tissue oxygen tension: a review. *Undersea & hyperbaric medicine*. 1998 Oct 1;25(3):179.

[51] Niinikoski J. Oxygen and wound healing. *Clin. Plast. Surg*. 1977; 4: 361-374.

[52] Rosenberg J (1995) Late postoperative hypoxemia. Mechanisms and clinical implications. *These. Dan. Med. Bull.* 42 40–461.

[53] Hecht S S. Research opportunities related to establishing standards for tobacco products under the Family Smoking Prevention and Tobacco Control Act. *Nicotine Tob. Res.* 2012;14:18–28

[54] Yang G P, Longaker T (2003) Abstinence from smoking reduces incisional infection: a randomized controlled trial (Editorial). *Ann. Surg*. 238:6–8.

[55] Jensen J A, Goodson W H, Hopf H W, Hunt T K. Cigarette smoking decreases tissue oxygen. *Archives of surgery*. 1991 Sep 1;126(9):1131-4.

[56] Jorgensen L N, Kallehave F, Christensen E, Siana JE, Gottrup F. Less collagen production in smokers. *Surgery*. 1998 Apr 1;123(4):450-5.

[57] Aicher A, Rentsch M, Sasaki K I, Ellwart J W, Fändrich F, Siebert R, Cooke J P, Dimmeler S, Heeschen C. Nonbone marrow-derived circulating progenitor cells contribute to postnatal neovascularization following tissue ischemia. Circulation research. 2007 Mar 2;100(4):581-9.

[58] Grant Marianne A. Aly Karsan, in *Hematology* (Seventh Edition), 2018.

[59] Carmeliet P. Mechanisms of angiogenesis and arteriogenesis. *Nature Medicine*. 2000;6(4):389–395. DOI: 10.1038/74651.

[60] Eliceiri B. P., Paul R., Schwartzberg P. L., Hood J. D., Leng J., Cheresh D. A. Selective requirement for Src kinases during VEGF-induced angiogenesis and vascular permeability. *Molecular Cell*. 1999;4(6):915–924. doi: 10.1016/s1097-2765(00)80221-x.

[61] Ribatti D. The involvement of endothelial progenitor cells in tumor angiogenesis. *J. Cell Mol. Med.* 2004;8(3):294-300.

[62] Eliceiri B. P., Cheresh D. A. The role of αv integrins during angiogenesis: insights into potential mechanisms of action and clinical development. *Journal of Clinical Investigation.* 1999;103(9):1227–1230. DOI: 10.1172/jci6869.

[63] Conway E. M., Collen D., Carmeliet P. Molecular mechanisms of blood vessel growth. *Cardiovascular Research.* 2001;49(3):507–521. doi: 10.1016/s0008-6363(00)00281-9.

[64] Shweiki D, Itin A, Soffer D, Keshet E. Vascular endothelial growth factor induced by hypoxia may mediate hypoxia-initiated angiogenesis. *Nature.* 1992 Oct 29;359(6398):843-5.

[65] Semenza GL. HIF-1 and human disease: one highly involved factor. *Genes & development.* 2000 Aug 15;14(16):1983-91.

[66] Semenza G. L. Life with oxygen. *Science.* 2007;318(5847):62–64. DOI: 10.1126/science.1147949.

[67] Ema M., Taya S., Yokotani N., Sogawa K., Matsuda Y., Fujii-Kuriyama Y. A novel bHLH-PAS factor with close sequence similarity to hypoxia-inducible factor 1α regulates the VEGF expression and is potentially involved in lung and vascular development. *Proceedings of the National Academy of Sciences of the United States of America.* 1997;94(9):4273–4278. doi: 10.1073/pnas.94.9.4273.

[68] Park J. E., Keller G.-A., Ferrara N. The vascular endothelial growth factor (VEGF) isoforms: differential deposition into the subepithelial extracellular matrix and bioactivity of extracellular matrix-bound VEGF. *Molecular Biology of the Cell.* 1993;4(12):1317–1326. DOI: 10.1091/mbc.4.12.1317.

[69] Ben-Yosef Y., Miller A., Shapiro S., Lahat N. Hypoxia of endothelial cells leads to MMP-2-dependent survival and death. *The American Journal of Physiology—Cell Physiology.* 2005;289(5):C1321–C1331. DOI: 10.1152/ajpcell.00079.2005.

[70] Keely S, Glover L E, MacManus C F, Campbell E L, Scully M M, Furuta G T, Colgan S P. Selective induction of integrin β1 by hypoxia-inducible factor: implications for wound healing. *The FASEB Journal.* 2009 May;23(5):1338.

[71] Novosel EC, Kleinhans C, Kluger PJ. Vascularization is the key challenge in tissue engineering. *Advanced drug delivery reviews.* 2011 Apr 30;63(4-5):300-11.

[72] Lovett M, Lee K, Edwards A, Kaplan D L. Vascularization strategies for tissue engineering. *Tissue Eng. Part B Rev.* 2009 Sep;15(3):353-70. DOI: 10.1089/ten.TEB.2009.0085. PMID: 19496677; PMCID: PMC2817665.

[73] Oh S H, Ward C L, Atala A, Yoo J J, Harrison BS. Oxygen-generating scaffolds for enhancing engineered tissue survival. *Biomaterials.* 2009 Feb;30(5):757-62. DOI: 10.1016/j.biomaterials.2008.09.065. Epub 2008 Nov 18. PMID: 19019425.

[74] Bland E, Dréau D, Burg K J. Overcoming hypoxia to improve tissue-engineering approaches to regenerative medicine. *J. Tissue Eng. Regen. Med.* 2013 Jul;7(7):505-14. DOI: 10.1002/term.540. Epub 2012 Jul 4. PMID: 22761177.

[75] Barwinska D, Traktuev D O, Merfeld-Clauss S, Cook T G, Lu H, Petrache I, March KL. Cigarette Smoking Impairs Adipose Stromal Cell Vasculogenic Activity and Abrogates Potency to Ameliorate Ischemia. *Stem Cells.* 2018 Jun;36(6):856-867. doi: 10.1002/stem.2813. Epub 2018 Mar 28. PMID: 29589872; PMCID: PMC 5992062.

[76] McMurtrey, Richard J. "Multi-compartmental biomaterial scaffolds for patterning neural tissue organoids in models of neurodevelopment and tissue regeneration." *Journal of Tissue Engineering* 7 (2016): 2041731416671926.

[77] Semenza, Gregg L. "Life with oxygen." *Science* 318.5847 (2007): 62-64.

[78] Newland H, Eigel D, Rosser A E, Werner C, Newland B. Oxygen producing microscale spheres affect cell survival in conditions of oxygen-glucose deprivation in a cell specific manner: implications for cell transplantation. *Biomaterials science*. 2018;6(10):2571-7.

Chapter 3

Vascular Development, Its Genetic Control and Effects on Diseases

Ugur Gumus*, MD
Department of Medical Genetics, Gaziantep Dr. Ersin Arslan Training and Research Hospital, Gaziantep, Turkey

Abstract

Knowledge of genetics and its role in diseases is rapidly increasing. Chronic diseases, cardiovascular pathologies, and cancer have a strong genetic background. A thorough understanding of the role of genetics opens up new possibilities for the prevention and treatment of these conditions. One stepstone of this understanding is the genetic pathways of vascular development and their effect on disease progression. Strict genetic paths control vasculogenesis and angiogenesis. Initially, these processes were believed to occur only in embryonic life; however, recent studies showed they also occur in adult tissues. The continuation of vascular development in adult tissues shows that vascularization can effectively treat chronic diseases. This chapter will try to explain the genetic control of vascular development in both embryonal and adult life and discuss new tools for diagnosing, preventing, and treating diseases in light of the knowledge of these processes.

Keywords: vasculogenesis, angiogenesis, vascular development, genetic control, embryonic life

---

* Corresponding Author's Email: uurgumusmd@gmail.com.

In: Vascularization and Its Role in Medicine and Tissue Engineering
Editors: Emre Bulbul and Murat Oguz Ozilhan
ISBN: 979-8-89113-041-8

Introduction

The cardiovascular system is the first functional organ system that develops in the human embryo [1]. Vasculogenesis is the de novo formation process of blood vessels that arise from blood islands (described below). On the other hand, angiogenesis is sprouting new vessels from existing ones. In almost all vertebrate embryos, vasculogenesis and hematopoiesis begin in the yolk sac (a membranous sac attached to an embryo, formed by cells of the hypoblast adjacent to the bilaminar embryonic disc), which plays a role in embryonic circulation. The yolk sac is formed by mesodermal cells that migrate into the extra-embryonic region after gastrulation. This results in a two-layered tissue, neighboring extra-embryonic mesoderm and primitive endoderm. This interaction between two germ lines is essential for the initiation of hematopoiesis. At the end of gastrulation, the yolk sac contains primitive erythroid cells and vascular endothelial cells called "blood islands."

Blood islands are the earliest structures of the cardiovascular system in early embryonal development [2]. The first blood islands appear in the mesoderm surrounding the yolk sac wall at three weeks of development and slightly later in the lateral plate mesoderm and other regions. The fusion of blood islands results in forming the primary vascular plexus. After the first week of embryonal development vascular plexus begins to form. The area vasculosa (vascularized part of the yolk sac) is concordant with the mesodermal layer. The cells which form the blood islands are called hemangioblasts. These cells are the vessels' endothelial cells' progenitors, which are angioblasts and hematopoietic cells. Except for the edges of the lateral yolk sac mesoderm and sinus rhomboidalis (embryonic tail), all of the yolk sac has primordial vascular cells [3]. Mesoderm cells adjacent to visceral endoderm are the precursor of hemangioblasts and the first hematopoietic cells of the embryo. Hemangioblasts located in the center of the blood islands form hematopoietic stem cells. However, the peripheral ones are the precursors of blood vessels.

Angiogenesis starts after the formation of the dorsal aorta and cardinal veins [4]. Arteries, veins, and lymphatic system specification occur after angioblast induction. During the fourth and fifth weeks of development, each pharyngeal arch has its cranial nerve and artery. In the fifth week of development, the vitelline veins (vessels carrying blood from the yolk sac to the sinus venosus), umbilical veins (originates from chorionic villi), and cardinal veins are the three pairs of major veins that can be identified. Lastly, the lymphatic system begins developing after the cardiovascular system is not appearing until the fifth week of development. Lymphatic veins develop from the endothelium of veins [5].

We can see that blood and vascular structure cells are developed from the same progenitor cell group. Vascular and blood cells are differentiated from mesoderm. Differentiation of the tissue is determined before the gastrulation stage [6]. Unlike gastrointestinal and respiratory epithelia, the endothelium is developed from mesoderm [7]. But this process starts with the signals from the visceral endoderm.

- One of these signals is the Indian hedgehog signaling molecule (IHH) [3], which induces the formation of hemangioblasts. IHH is one signal that commits multipotent mesodermal cells to endothelial cell lineage. This signal also plays a part in the development of neural ectoderm. In addition, some recent data shows that IHH expression from visceral endoderm is sufficient to induce hematopoiesis and vasculogenesis in the early gastrulation stage [8].
- Other important molecules are transforming growth factor-beta (TGF-beta), like factors that induce mesoderm formation [9]. Mainly, activins induce mesoderm development, especially muscle precursors. Even though this signaling path is related to mesodermal differentiation, it is not directly intertwined with vasculogenesis. But the activin pathway (includes SMAD2, NODAL, and SMAD3) has a part in transforming mesodermal cell lineage to early muscle cells. This muscle tissue joins with the late development of blood vessels [10]. Some animal data shows activin is also a participant in epidermis and notochord development.
- Bone morphogenic protein 4 (BMP4) is also essential for mesoderm differentiation [11] and a part of the TGF-beta superfamily of polypeptide signaling molecules. Its conservation between species points out that BMP4 plays a crucial role in embryonal development. In other embryonic tissues (tooth bud, limb bud), BMP4 expression has been detected [12]. BMP4 expression in embryonic stem cells enhances the differentiation of hematopoietic cells. Also, for the cardiovascular system, cardiac muscle formation is mediated by both activin-A and BMP4. Also, this shows that these molecules are part of embryonic heart development, not only in vasculogenesis [13]. There is some evidence in animal studies that BMP4 might also be a downstream effector of IHH.

- Some recent data suggest that fibroblast growth factor (FGF) signaling is required for the induction of paraxial mesoderm but not for axial mesoderm [14]. Mainly, this pathway is essential for cell migration during gastrulation. Thus mesoderm formation includes significant cell migration, and FGF signaling is crucial to this development. Some early data suggests that overexpression of the FGF path suppresses blood island formation and works against BMP4 signaling [15]. This data also suggests that FGF4 restricts mesoderm proportion to form blood while promoting myogenesis. For early aspects of myogenesis, FGF signaling has been shown as essential recently [16]. But, some recent data shows that FGF4 controls the degree of hematopoiesis, not only repressing it. It also suggests that FGF4 is essential for correct blood and skeletal muscle cell lineage specification [17]. Also, FGF2 induces blood island development through FGFR2 from hemangioblasts [18]. Synergistic signaling between IHH and FGF2 is thought to promote the expression of the vascular endothelial-derived growth factor (VEGF) receptor KDR (also known as FLK1 or VEGFR2) in adjacent mesodermal cells. A role for FGF2 in forming endothelial precursors, angioblasts, from mesoderm has been demonstrated, where explant cultures consisting of only mesoderm cannot undergo angioblast formation unless treated with FGF2 [19]. It seems that the critical role of FGF2 during vascular induction is the upregulation of the kinase insert domain receptor (KDR).
- The VEGF pathway is critical in embryonic vasculogenesis and angiogenesis [20]. VEGF production starts mainly from endodermal cells and, unlike the other molecules mentioned above, does not play a role in mesoderm formation. VEGF's main effect starts after the formation of mesoderm and developing endothelial structure and differentiation. As we can see now, these molecules work coherently to develop the precursor of the vascular cells. VEGF has essential properties characteristic of a potential regulator of embryonic angiogenesis and endothelial cell functions [17]. VEGF is a selective mitogen for endothelial cells. Therefore, it is an essential factor in angiogenesis. KDR and FMS-Related Tyrosine Kinase 1 (FLT1-also called VEGFR1) is also essential in vasculogenesis. KDR binds VEGF with high affinity in vitro and is expressed early in development by endothelial cell precursors [21]. Interaction between endothelial cells, pericytes, and vascular smooth muscle (mural cells)

is crucial for vascular development and maintenance. Endothelial cells arise from KDR-expressing (KDR+) mesoderm cells, whereas mural cells are believed to derive from mesoderm, neural crest, or epicardial cells and migrate to form the vessel wall. VEGF promotes endothelial cell differentiation, whereas mural cells are induced by platelet-derived growth factor-BB (PDGFB) [22]. FLT1 is a regulator receptor for VEGF activity, and KDR controls mitogenic endothelial activity [23]. Recent data informs us about two novel VEGF receptors: Neuropilin (NRP1 and NRP2). They are expressed initially in the nervous system but also in endothelial cells. Animal studies suggest that both receptors have a role in the structure and organization of blood vessels [24]. VEGF signaling is also essential for capillary plexus formation. Vascular remodeling and endothelial cell proliferation are controlled by both inducer and inhibitor signals. As previously described, FGF2 and VEGF are needed to induce endothelial cell proliferation. Also, retinaldehyde dehydrogenase 2 (RALDH2-also expressed in visceral endoderm) and TGF-beta-1 work as anti-proliferative signals to repress uncontrollable vascular development [25].

Other molecules that join the mesoderm formation, blood island differentiation, the fusion of blood islands and endothelial cell differentiation, and primary capillary plexus formation are fibronectin, platelet-endothelial cell adhesion molecule, laminin, type IV collagen, and VE-cadherin.

Angiogenesis

This process is the formation of blood vessels from already existing ones, including two different stages: sprouting of endothelial cells and vessel lumen separation. The importance of angiogenesis is that thanks to this process, other germ layer-originated tissues too vascularized by angiogenesis. The first stage of angiogenesis is the sprouting process. New capillary forms from small venules from other vessels. This is followed by basement membrane degradation executed by enzymes such as collagenase. Then, endothelial cells migrate to angiogenic stimuli. Mitosis of these cells progresses away from the sprouting origin, ensuring the connection of distinct sprouts and loop formation. Flow begins after that and is followed by smooth muscle alignment with endothelial cells, and a new basement membrane is formed [26].

The second phase of angiogenesis is vessel lumen separation, also called "intussusceptive microvascular growth" (IMG). From the vessel wall, a new lumen will be formed from the endothelial layer retreats. This results in the elongation of the vessel lumen around a unit of interstitial tissue called the pillar core in the vessel wall. Collagen fibrils join the formation of this core. This pillar separates itself from the lateral vessel wall by thinning the endothelial cells. This forms a ring and allows for the newly formed vessel lumen's expansion. It is followed by the reorganization of the endothelial junctions to allow an increasing number of endothelial cells to take part in the pillar lining, which is also a prerequisite for subsequent pillar growth. Collagen fiber synthesis is required for this pillar core's stabilization. Peri-endothelial cells might be responsible for collagen production, especially type 1. In adult tissue repair or tumor angiogenesis, these peri-endothelial cells that express endothelial-specific markers migrate toward blood vessel walls and form a lamella around endothelial cells. Flow is not deterred during this process, and a basement membrane is finally formed [27].

Molecular regulation of these processes explains the genes responsible for angiogenesis in adult life, and some of them are also essential factors for vascular effects on disease progression. The molecular regulation of angiogenesis is the regulation of distinct steps.

- The VEGF is also responsible for regulating angiogenesis, similar to its role in vasculogenesis. A cell group called circulating endothelial progenitor cell (EPC) is discovered in adult angiogenesis, and it is shown that VEGF stimulation adds them to endothelial cell markers [28]. Like circulating EPCs, resident EPCs reside in the endothelial intima of large vessels. These cells are ready to proliferate in response to tissue injury. These cells expressing the CD34 antigen can transdifferentiate into mature EPCs and form tubule formation in arterial rings [29]. Sprouting angiogenesis is characterized by sprouts composed of endothelial cells, which usually grow toward VEGF stimulus. Most types of parenchymal cells respond to a hypoxic environment by secreting VEGF. There do not appear to be redundant growth factor mechanisms that can replace the role of VEGF-A in hypoxia-induced angiogenesis. Long, thin cellular processes on tip cells called filopodia secrete large amounts of proteolytic enzymes, which digest a pathway through the extracellular matrix for the developing sprout. The filopodia of tip cells are heavily endowed with VEGF-A receptors. When a sufficient number of filopodia on a given tip cell have anchored to the substratum, contraction of actin filaments within the filopodia pulls the tip cell toward the VEGF-A stimulus [30]. VEGF also stimulates DLL4 expression, which binds to its receptor on neighboring cells. This ensures sprouting formation. VEGF also plays a role in IMG, but other transcription factors have a part too. VEGF plays this part via its receptors KDR and FLT1. While the KDR receptor is dominant during early vasculogenesis, FLT1 is prominent during the remodeling of the primary vascular plexus and subsequent angiogenesis.

- A group of molecules called angiopoietins have receptors predominantly expressed on endothelial cells [31]. These receptors are called tyrosine kinase with immunoglobulin and EGF factor homology domain (TIE1 and TIE2). The detailed analysis of TIE2 receptor-deficient embryos revealed malformations of the heart derived from a lack of interaction between the endocardium and myocardium. Abnormally large vessels were detected in the extraembryonic yolk sac circulation and many vascular networks throughout the embryo. It seems that lack of angiopoietin stimuli causes a failure of endothelial cell interaction with their extracellular matrix and a recruitment deficit of peri-endothelial cells. This causes the collapse of vascular segments due to the aberrant morphology of tissue pillars [32]. According to recent data angiopoietin system mainly supports the IMG rather than sprouting. Angiopoietin (ANG)-1 is weakly mitogenic for endothelial cells, so it does not cause endothelial cell proliferation or tube formation but is chemotactic for endothelial cells [33]. It also stabilizes plexus formation, increases the survival of networks, and prevents apoptotic death [34]. Working with VEGF enhances the capillary density and luminal diameter of vessels. ANG-2 does not affect TIE2, instead blocks the ANG1 activity. On the other hand, ANG2 is coexpressed with VEGF, leading us to believe that it has a role in endothelial sprouting. The TIE1 receptor tyrosine kinase has been initially implicated with a survival function for endothelial cells and a stabilization effect on the vessel wall. Animal studies show that TIE1 activity deficiency results in "hyperactive" endothelial cells and demonstrate TIE1 receptor could be an inhibitor of angiogenesis [35].
- Another receptor tyrosine kinase family, Ephrin-B receptors, and their ligands called ephrins have been shown to induce embryonic angiogenesis. Studies show that arterial and venous sites are at least

partly genetically determined before the typical physiological characteristics have developed. There are two subtypes of these receptors. Ephrin-B2 is strictly located on arterial endothelial cells, whereas Ephrin-B4 marked only venous endothelial cells. It seems this separation has a role in selecting vessel fate, whether it is going to be an artery or vena, and remodeling the primary plexus [36].

Some other factors that have a part in angiogenesis are connexin 45, matrix metalloproteinases, the Notch family, and integrins.

Hematopoiesis

As previously mentioned, the first hematopoietic cells of embryonic life are present in the yolk sac. The yolk sac forms a two-layered structure consisting of visceral endoderm and mesoderm. The first morphological evidence of hematopoiesis is the pools of immature erythroid cells within the yolk sac. These so-called "blood islands" consist of primitive erythroid cells enveloped by endothelial cells. Blood islands cell groups differentiate into both endothelial cell lineage and hematopoietic progenitors. Both cell lines have a common progenitor called hemangioblasts. Primitive hematopoiesis is initiated as two waves in the blood islands, producing primitive macrophages and primitive erythrocytes, thus providing the developing embryos with oxygen and their first line of defense against pathogens [37]. At the end of the first week of intrauterine life, primitive hematopoiesis is initiated in the yolk sac. This is only the first wave. The second wave is in the second week, when definitive hematopoietic stem cells, arise in the aorta-gonad-mesonephros (AGM) region. Within this region, precursor cells of hematopoiesis are observed as clumps of cells on the walls of the newly formed dorsal aorta, and umbilical and vitelline arteries [38]. 7th day of embryonic life, a few primitive erythroid cells are detectable. Next 24 hours, these cells start to express fetal hemoglobin. Other hematopoietic progenitors are also produced, including macrophage and megakaryocyte progenitors in the early yolk sac. This 24 hours development is called primitive hematopoiesis. The definitive hematopoiesis process starts with the progenitors that show the same morphology, stick to the same lineage, and express similar gene pathways with mature hematopoietic development cells from bone marrow and fetal liver. The definitive hematopoiesis can be observed on the 9th day of embryonic life [39]. These progenitor cells arising in the AGM region begin the circulation and migrate to the fetal liver on the 10th day of development. The fetal liver will be the predominant hematopoiesis site until just before birth, when circulating stem cells become seeded at the spleen and bone marrow.

Apart from the common origin of is hemangioblast idea, there are two other observations. One is that blood-forming cells are specified from the endothelium, known as hemogenic endothelium. From FLK-1 positive hemangioblast, hemogenic endothelial intermediate cell emerges, and after that, hematopoietic fate continues. As mentioned above, hematopoiesis precursors clustered on the walls of primitive vascular structures support this inference. The fact that the timing of the two different cell specializations is the same seems to be supportive. In a study, primitive endothelial cells were isolated from human embryonic stem cell cultures. These cells express the endothelial markers but not the hematopoietic lineage marker CD45. Under the VEGF effect, these cells were shown to differentiate to mature endothelial cells. However, treatment with hematopoietic growth factors results in hematopoietic development [40]. This information shows us that hematopoietic and endothelial differentiation occurs as a hierarchical organization of cell fate commitment. The other idea about the origin of blood cells is that hematopoietic progenitors may be independently specified during gastrulation. This idea suggests that there is no typical ancestor cell of both lineages, but instead, they are specified independently during gastrulation. Studies show that different stages of primitive embryo cells contribute to different cell lineages. Cells derived from the primitive streak preferentially contribute to the erythrocyte precursor population of the developing vascular blood islands.

Cells derived from the primitive streak of mid-primitive streak-stage embryos appear to contribute primarily to the endothelium. These observations suggest that early progenitor cells are recruited to both lineages at different gastrulation stages [41]. Regardless of the source of the cells, our data is abundant on molecules that provide genetic control of hematopoiesis.

- The VEGF/KDR pathway plays a crucial role in the regulation of hematopoiesis as well as vasculogenesis. As previously described in the vasculogenesis section, KDR is an early antigenic marker of developing endothelial cells. But also, animal studies show KDR-deficient embryos fail to develop hematopoietic cells [42]. This suggests that VEGF signaling from the yolk sac endoderm is required to differentiate mesoderm to erythroid cell lineage. Deficient VEGF activity in animal embryos fails vasculogenesis and hematopoiesis

[43]. This signal path may not be essential for the initial specification of precursor erythroid cells. Some data shows that development is impaired, but precursor cell count is not deficient when VEGF expression is insufficient [44]. It leads us to VEGF/KDR signaling is required for survival, migration, and clonal expansion of hematopoietic progenitors rather than specification.

- Another essential factor is TAL1 (also known as Stem Cell Leukemia Hematopoietic Transcription Factor-SCL). TAL1 is first expressed during embryo development with KDR in visceral endoderm and initiates mesoderm differentiation into the hematopoietic cell lineage [45]. TAL1 is required to generate both primitive and definitive hematopoietic lineages and to remodel the yolk sac vascularization.
- GATA1 and 2 are transcription factors essential in determining the hematopoietic lineage. For example, animal embryo studies with GATA1 deficient tissue show termination of erythroid differentiation [46]. On the other hand, GATA2 loss causes primary to detect in primitive hematopoiesis [47].
- RUNT-Related Transcription Factor 1 (RUNX1) is another essential transcription factor for definitive hematopoiesis. RUNX1 deficiency results in normal yolk sac hematopoiesis but the failure of definitive hematopoiesis [48]. In addition, RUNX1 seems to support the specification of hemogenic endothelium (endothelium cells that can be transformed into hematopoietic precursor cells; look above), which contributes to definitive hematopoiesis [49].
- LMO2 is another transcription factor required for vascular development and yolk sac hematopoiesis. LMO2 might function cooperatively with GATA1 and TAL1 to specification erythroid cells [50].
- The platelet glycoprotein receptor IIb/IIIa is formed with two proteins; CD41 and CD61. This protein complex was considered a platelet-specific-receptor and phenotypic marker for the platelet lineage. But, some recent data shows that CD41 expression is not limited to platelet lineage, and also may serve as a marker for the onset of definitive hematopoiesis in the embryo and in embryonic stem cell-derived hematopoietic cells in vitro [51]. More data demonstrate that CD41 expression on the first hematopoietic progenitor cells persists from the primitive and definitive hematopoiesis to fetal liver and adult bone marrow. One role the

CD41/61 receptor may play is in the interaction of the progenitor cells with extracellular matrix molecules in the yolk sac [52]. In addition, more recent studies indicate CD41 may act as an organizing molecule for adhesion to fibronectin and basal membrane-derived stroma [53].

A Brief Summary of Heart Development

We are not going to discuss the details of the embryologic development of the heart in detail, but briefly explain to identify the key elements of genetic control of it.

The mammalian heart is a highly modified vessel developing from a simple tube to a pump under electrical and endocrine control. Cardiac development can be divided into overlapping phases such as mesoderm formation, specification of cardiac progenitor cells, differentiation of cardiac cell types, formation of the heart tube, and chamber formation and maturation. These phases include two different cell sources: the primary heart field and the secondary heart field. Myocardial cells are derivated from mesoderm, which emerges from the primitive streak during gastrulation. The cells then extend across the midline to form a crescent-shaped epithelium, the cardiac crescent, which fuses at the midline to form the early heart tube. The heart tube undergoes looping and is shaped by this process and expansion of the myocardium. The primary heart field begins to form during 16 to 18 days of embryonic life. This will be the significant part of the left ventricle, atrium, and right ventricle. The remaining parts of the heart come from a secondary heart field which begins to form during 20 to 21 days of the embryonal life. This cell comes from the splanchnic mesoderm. Like vasculogenesis, neighboring pharyngeal endoderm induces the primary heart field to begin the formation of an endothelial-lined tube surrounded by myoblasts. This tube elongates as cells are added from the secondary heart field. On day 23 cardiac tube begins to bend to organize by regions along its craniocaudal axis. This process results in the formation of conotruncus, and then primitive trabeculae begin to form. This formation is in the early stages of the atriums and ventricles [2]. A critical part of heart development is the septation of the primitive tube into four chambers with different roles. The growth, differentiation, and specialization of muscles, valves, and conduction tissue follow it. By the 13th day of embryonic life, the heart already contains four chambers coordinating blood flow through the pulmonary and systemic circulation. However, genetic control of this process is not as strict as vasculogenesis. All the factors below are optional for heart development, but some insufficiency results in incoordination of formation and heart defects.

- It seems that NK2 homeobox 5 (NKX2-5) (also called cardiac-specific homeobox 1-CSX) is working with T-Box transcription factor 5 (TBX5) to bind to the promoter of the gene encoding cardiac-specific natriuretic peptide precursor type A (NPPA). This induction requires the secretion of BMP2-4 and FGFs secreted and the activity of wingless-related integration site (WNT) proteins which prevent the initiation of heart development inhibited. The combination of these two causes the expression of NKX2-5, the maestro of cardiac development [54]. Inhibition of WNT proteins is executed by WNT inhibitory factor 1 (WIN1). Also, NKX2-5 upregulates the expression of heart-and neural crest derivatives expressed 1-2 (HAND1 and HAND2). They are both transcription factors expressed in the primitive heart tube and contribute to the expansion and differentiation of the ventricles [55, 56].
- Following the mesoderm formation, cardiogenic precursor cells are differentiated by the mesoderm posterior essential helix-loop-helix transcription factor 1 (MESP1) expression [57]. The earliest molecular markers for cardiac progenitors, the transcription factors MESP1 and MESP2, are expressed transiently in newly formed mesoderm at the primitive-streak stage [58]. More recently, it has been shown that MESP1+ cardiovascular progenitors are distinct and required for the exit from the pluripotent state and the induction of the cardiovascular gene expression process. Animal studies show that MESP1 expression identifies the necessity of distinction of different cell lineage and regional segregation of heart development [59]. MESP1 upregulates the genes of both heart fields and, at the same time, inhibits other pathways. Expression of MESP1 and 2 seems t mark both myocardial cell lineages (primary and secondary).
- After the formation of the cardiac tube, the venous portion is specified by retinoic acid (RA). RA is produced by the mesoderm that neighbors the sinus venosus and atrium. The expression of retinaldehyde dehydrogenase follows RA exposure so that these cells can produce their RA. It is shown in animal data that RA production from ventricular precursors is essential for the correct specification of the ventricles and sino-atrial tissues. RA's effect on the sino-atrial

tissue seems coordinated by the human alkaline phosphatase reporter gene (HAP). Both excess and insufficiency of RA cause cardiac anomalies during cardiogenesis [60]. Also, anteroposterior patterning (AP) is affected by RA expression too.

- Some transcription factors express only in embryonic heart development, and some are restricted to specific tissues. For example, TBX5 is only expressed in the primary heart field, while FGF8, TBX 1, FOXC1/2, and islet (ISL) 1 are specific to secondary heart field determination [54]. GATA4/5/6 are other transcription factors in the regulation of cardiac development. As we previously see, GATA1-3 are essential regulators of hematopoietic stem cells, whereas GATA4-6 are expressed in various mesoderm and endoderm-originated tissue. GATA4 is one of the earliest molecules in developing heart cells and continues this expression throughout life. GATA5 is only expressed in embryonic life, and GATA6 is expressed during embryonic and fetal development of multiple systems, including heart, pulmonary, gastrointestinal, and urogenital regions. It seems that GATA4 insufficiency fails heart tube formation and indicates that expression of GATA4 appears indispensable for proper endodermal differentiation and ventral morphogenesis, but not necessarily for differentiation of cardiac myocytes. The conserved GATA6 transcription factor is an early marker of the cardiogenic lineage. GATA6 participates in forming the definitive atrioventricular (AV) conduction system and developing the endocardial cushions of the AV canal [61].
- TBX family is particular to cardiac development, and most insufficiency results in severe cardiac defects. One of these factors, TBX5, may be involved in AP patterning or morphogenesis linked to RA signaling [62]. TBX5 is required for the formation of the posterior heart [63]. It is shown that TBX1 is essential for valve septation and separation of the aorta and pulmonary artery. Deletion of TBX1 is the main aspect of cardiac anomalies seen in 22 q deletion syndrome and represents an overview of its role in cardiogenesis. The same data shows that overflow tract development (vascular conduit that connects the embryonic right ventricle to the aortic sac) is TBX1 dependent, but not for myocyte and endothelial cells for this region. In the secondary heart field, TBX1 expression is a downstream effect of the NXK2-5 function [64].

- The final transformation is regulated by a set of differentiation genes, such as the myosin light chain and heavy chain encoding the structural proteins. Endoderm-originated factors continue to influence cardiogenesis during all of the development. BMP2, Dickopf WNT signaling pathway inhibitor 1 (DKK1), ISL1, TBX1, and FGF8 are some of the signals expressed by endodermal tissue that joins the cardiogenesis. ISL1 is particularly important for making cardiac progenitors contribute to the heart. One progenitor population expresses ISL1 and will give rise to the outflow tract, right ventricle, a subset of left ventricular cells, and, surprisingly, a large number of atrial cells. The other does not express ISL1 and will give rise to the most left ventricle and atrial cells. It is also required for the proliferation of the outflow tract, right ventricle, and most of the atrial progenitors [65]. Just like WIN1, DKK1 is another WNT pathway inhibitor. WNT proteins can activate some pathways that regulate proper cardiogenesis tightly. This regulation depends on a specific control of WNT pathways and timely inhibition of their activity. ISL1 acts upstream of DKK1. Loss of DKK1 does not alter mesoderm formation or cardiac specification but affects the normal differentiation process of cardiomyocytes [66].

The other factors that participate the heart development are FGF10, which contributes to myocardium development; paired-like homeodomain transcription factor 2 (PITX2), which contributes to symmetrical development and looping of the heart; fork-head box P4 (FOXP4), which ensure the two distinct heart field's fusion, myocyte enhancer factor 2C (MEF2C) which contributes to cardiomyocyte differentiation. TBX20 participates with myocardial hypertrophy, and lack of expression results in abnormal myocardial chambers. TBX20 also synergizes with ISL1 and GATA4 to activate the MEF2C and NKX2-5 [67].

We are not going to discuss congenital cardiac anomalies and cardiomyopathies or muscle diseases that affect cardiac muscle too here. These conditions are primarily genetic disorders but do not interact with the vascularization process and are out of the context of this chapter.

Vascular Formation in Trauma and Diseases

Blood vessel growth occurs in response to both physiological and pathological stimuli. Hypoxia is a significant stimulus for the expansion of the vascular bed. When tissues grow beyond the oxygenation limit, hypoxia triggers some signals for new vessel formation. This is part of physiological angiogenesis. Physiological angiogenesis occurs in response to exercise to accommodate the active tissue's increased oxygen and metabolic demands. Hypoxia-inducible transcription factors (HIFs) upregulate many angiogenic genes discussed in the chapter. HIFs are heterodimeric transcription factors. Just like hemoglobin, they have alfa and beta subunits too. The HIF-1a subunit is continually synthesized and degraded within adequately perfused cells with normal oxygenation. Under hypoxia, however, subunits are stabilized and form heterodimers with HIF-1beta, which is not subject to oxygen-dependent regulation [68]. HIF-1a is necessary and sufficient for the hypoxia-induced expression of multiple angiogenic growth factors, including VEGF, placental growth factor (PLGF), ANG1, ANG2, and PDGFB [69]. HIF1 also has some intracellular endothelial roles. It regulates the expression of VEGFR1 and the migration of migrating stem cells towards VEGF and PLGF stimuli. It might also implicate stromal-derived growth factor 1 (SDF1) expression and CXCR4, which is the SDF1 receptor. HIFs also activate phosphoglycerate kinase (PGK) and erythropoietin (EPO). PGK increases glycolysis, and EPO activates erythropoiesis. Some well-known molecules modulate HIF expression; epidermal growth factor (EGF), insulin, insulin-like growth factor (IGF)-1 and 2, angiotensin II, thrombin, PDGF-B, interleukin (IL)1B, tumor necrosis factor (TNF)-alfa, and heregulin. Regardless of oxygen level, p53 mediates HIF degradation, although prolonged hypoxia activates p53 [70]. Big mitogen-activated protein kinase (BMK)1 is another negative regulator of HIF1 stability independent from oxygen level.

Under normal circumstances, cells are adapted to perform their physiological functions under relatively low oxygen levels, often referred to as physiological hypoxia. Tissue oxygen levels may be further reduced than the physiological limit due to rapid oxygen consumption and poor circulation. The imbalance between O2 supply and demand leads to hypoxia, a physiological stimulus that induces cells to produce angiogenic cytokines such as VEGF. In minutes VEGF expression climbs to 30-fold. VEGF stimulates physiological and pathological angiogenesis, as described above [71]. VEGF does activate not only angiogenesis but also increases vascular permeability.

Hypoxia is not only a physiological process but may also be part of a pathological process. For example, when an artery is occluded, its vascular territory becomes ischemic. The arterial system often has collateral vessels so the ischemic region can be saved. Collateral need increases with sheer stress. Under stress, cells produce growth factors and proteinases, which enable muscle cells to migrate.

Cytokines such as monocyte chemoattractant protein (MCP19), TGF-beta1, TNF-alfa, and granulocyte-macrophage colony-stimulating factor (CSF) joins the fray and enhance collateral growth, while IL-10 is a inhibitory. PLGF is a VEGF form from the placenta that also enhances collateral growth via stimulating endothelial and muscle cell growth. If the main flow vessel is stenotic, new vessel formation by sprouting is not a solution to the problem. When the cause of the ischemia is stenosis of a large vessel, in addition to angiogenesis, vessel remodeling is required by increasing luminal diameter to increase blood flow for bypassing the stenosis part. SDF1 and PLGF help VEGF stimulate angiogenic cells' mobilization [72].

Along with VEGF, moderate hypoxia also promotes the expression of endothelial nitric oxide synthase. This increases flow and vascular permeability, so endothelial precursors and inflammatory cells can interact with tissue. Severe hypoxia, though, might cause endothelial and muscle cell apoptosis. Diabetic injuries are perfect examples of this process. Severe hypoxia in diabetic wounds fails to promote angiogenesis due to apoptotic cell death. Hyperbaric oxygen treatment pulls the tissue out of a low-oxygen environment so the tissue can trigger healthy angiogenesis [73]. Like endothelial cells, smooth muscle cells are part of significantly larger vessels than capillary ones. Cyclooxygenase (COX)2 and PDGF-beta are essential to smooth muscle proliferation. Hypoxic tissue promotes monocyte migration with many molecules, such as MCP1, CSF1, VEGF, SDF1, and TNF-alfa. Monocytes transform into macrophages when they arrive. Macrophages promote angiogenesis by secreting matrix metalloproteinases (MMP) and other factors such as VEGF, FGF2, IL2, and TNF-alfa [70].

Trauma to the blood vessel interrupts healthy blood flow and creates a hypoxic environment. This causes HIF stabilization and inflammatory cell infiltration [74]. Muscle ischemia also leads to HIF and other angiogenic factor activation. In addition, myeloid and endothelial progenitors are recruited to support angiogenesis in ischemic muscle. Overexpression of HIF1 promotes and reduces infarct region size in the myocardium in animal studies [75]. In muscle tissue, HIF1 overexpression induces the expression of PLGF, PFGF-B, VEGF, SDF1, and MCP1.

Atherosclerosis is the primary cause of coronary artery disease and stroke. Mendelian disorders such as familial hypercholesterolemia, hypertriglyceridemia, and hyperlipoproteinemia have significantly increased coronary artery disease risk. Mutations of apolipoprotein C3 (ApoC3), angiopoietin-like 3 (ANGPTL3), apolipoprotein B (ApoB), proprotein convertase subtilisin/kexin type 9 (PCSK9), low-density lipoprotein R (LDLR), LDLRAP1, ApoA2, growth hormone R (GHR), LPL, glycosylphosphatidylinositol-anchored HDL binding protein 1 (GPIHBP1), ApoA5, ApoEA, cAMP-responsive element-binding protein 3 like 3 (CREB3L3) and glycerol-3-phosphate dehydrogenase 1 (GPD1) have been known to cause these conditions. PCSK9 protein combines with LDLR-LDL and transfers this complex to degradation. Mutations of this gene, especially the gain of function ones, increase the degradation and release of LDL and subsequently cause hyperlipidemia and, thus, atherosclerosis. In addition, maturity-onset diabetes of the young (MODY) and homocysteine cause increased vessel disease. Cystathionine beta synthase enzyme is responsible for converting homocysteine to cystathionine, and the inability of this causes a high level of homocysteine and endothelial damage. Genetic-origin hypertension too affects cardiovascular disease risk. 11-beta hydroxysteroid dehydrogenase, 11-beta hydroxylase, 17-alfa hydroxylase, MR, and ENAC gene mutations cause hypertension and increase vascular disease risk. But these conditions explain only a small percentage of disease susceptibility; some do not cause atherosclerosis [76]. Atherosclerosis is a progressive disease characterized by the accumulation of lipids and fibrous elements in the large arteries and a cause of endothelial injury. Shear stress on the endothelial wall, such as flow disturbance, causes increased permeability of macromolecules. LDL uptake and smooth muscle cell proliferation and infiltration of inflammatory cells thicken the vessel wall, further blocking the flow, increasing tissue hypoxia, and inducing angiogenesis. New capillary formation leads to more macrophage infiltration and plaque expansion [77]. Many molecules mediate the process of atherosclerosis formation. ApoB is responsible for carrying LDL to the subendothelial matrix. Following LDL undergoes some modifications. 12,15 lipoxygenase (LO), inducible nitric oxide synthase (iNOS), myeloperoxidase, and lipase are some of the responsible enzymes for that. LDL oxidation is the main stepstone of plaque development. Some of these modifying enzymes have a considerable effect on the process. Animal data shows that 15-LO enzyme deficiency diminishes atherosclerosis development. HDL is a protective figure from atherosclerosis with its antioxidant effect and removal effect of cholesterol from peripheral tissues. HDL performs with paraoxonase 1 enzyme for its antioxidant property, so it slows LDL oxidation. ApoA1 and platelet-activating factor-acetylhydrolase also have antioxidant effects. More oxidation means more inflammatory response. Some adhesion molecules help inflammatory cells make entry into the artery wall. Animal data shows that MCP1 or CCR2 deficiency has significantly reduced atherosclerosis activity. This path has a role in monocyte recruitment in atherosclerosis. CXCR (chemokine receptor)3, IL10, E and P-selectin, VLA4, vascular cell adhesion molecule 1, and interferon-gamma are other factors in migration and inflammatory cell recruitment. M-CSF stimulates the proliferation, differentiation, and survival of macrophages. Macrophages that devour oxidized LDL become foam cells. Scavenger receptors (SR)-A and CD36 are the scavenger receptors for macrophages to bind to LDL. ApoE and ATP-binding cassette(ABC)A1 protect against such development by secreting cholesterol from macrophages. Animal data shows that acyl-cholesterol acyl transferase deficiency prevents cholesterol storage and plaque formation. Macrophages and T lymphocytes secrete cytokines and growth factors for muscle cell migration and extracellular matrix production. CD40 and its ligand play a major part in developing advanced lesions. Hypertension and atherosclerosis have a relationship. Angiotensin II, just like immune system cells, stimulates muscle cell growth and extracellular matrix production. PDGF is also a potent mitogen for smooth muscle cells. Acute coronary syndrome depends on the vulnerability of the plaque. Thin fibrous caps on plaques tend to rupture. Factors that induce foam cell formation, inflammatory cell migration, and cytokine secretion also impact thrombosis risk. Other than these factors, some genes have a risk impact on cardiovascular disease. Myocyte Enhancer Factor 2A (MEF2A) is one of these genes. It has a role in muscle cell formation. It is known that mutations of MEF2A increase coronary artery disease risk by autosomal dominant inheritance pattern [78]. Low-density lipoprotein receptor-related protein 6 (LRP6) is another gene that encodes a member of the LDLR family and consists of cell surface proteins involved in receptor-mediated endocytosis of specific ligands [79]. LRP6 mutations are related to early coronary artery disease susceptibility. CD36 is another gene that may be responsible for modulating lipid metabolism and cardiovascular risk in Caucasians [80]. Insulin receptor substrate 1 is another gene that serves as a docking protein that binds and activates other signal transduction molecules after being phosphorylated on tyrosine by insulin receptor kinase. Its mutations may cause insulin resistance and type 2 diabetes mellitus and increase coronary artery disease. Other genes whose mutations are related to coronary artery disease are chemokine ligand 2 (CCL2), nitric oxide synthase-3 (NOS3), dual-specificity tyrosine-regulated kinase 1B (DYRK1B), junctional cadherin 5 associated (JCAD), and MMP3. Some structural anomalies might be related to coronary artery disease too. Several loci have been identified: CHDS1, mapped to 16pter-p13; CHDS2, mapped to 2q21.1-q22; CHDS3, mapped to Xq23-q26; CHDS4, mapped to 14q32; CHDS5, mapped to 3q13; CHDS8, mapped to 9p21; and CHDS9 mapped to 8p22. CHDS6 is associated with a polymorphism in the promoter region of the MMP3 gene, and CHDS7 represents susceptibility correlated with a common haplotype in the CD36 gene and high free fatty acid levels.

Premature infants are treated with oxygen for their lung condition, but sometimes, this results in retinopathy of prematurity (ROP). The provision of supplemental oxygen causes retinal hyperoxia, vasoconstriction, downregulation of VEGF, and the consequent cessation of normal retinal vascularisation. But metabolic demand and systemic factors with low vascularization cause retinal hypoxia. This time VEGF production is stimulated, leading to a renewal of vascularization. This might cause abnormal neovascularization. If the relative hypoxia did not damage tissue, normal vascularization could occur. We can see that VEGF up and downregulation is the main protagonist of this disease formation. But some recent animal data show that IGF binding protein (IGFP3) effectively recruits endothelial progenitor cells into retinal tissues [81]. Similarly, SDF1 plays a significant role in recruiting bone marrow-derived progenitor cells and contributes to pathological neovascularization [82].

Some rheumatologic diseases, such as rheumatoid arthritis, have vascularization problems. Inflammatory cells infiltrate the synovium, and the tissue becomes highly hypoxic due to the high metabolic rate. The high HIF levels cause this. In addition, HIF activates other angiogenic genes, ETS1, SDF1, and VEGF, which support angiogenesis in the synovium. This causes more infiltration, tissue mass, and, thus, more symptoms [83].

Hypoxia is a constant reality when cells are growing and multiplying incontrollable. Cancer cells require angiogenesis to grow. HIFs play significant roles in tumor vascularization. HIF1 deficiency has been shown to prevent vascularization in human gastric cancer [84]. Pro-angiogenic growth factors mainly activate surface receptors in paracrine and autocrine loops with the VEGF-A signaling. Despite the well-established master roles of VEGF signaling in literature, those processes are probably accomplished through a highly regulated interplay between VEGF and other pro-angiogenic factors.

HIF1-VEGF-VEGFR signaling path is a new targeting strategy for the treatment of cancer.

What Is the Difference between Physiologic Angiogenesis and Tumor Angiogenesis?

Tumor angiogenesis is a complete process. A balance of promoters and inhibitors regulates blood vessel growth. The balance of angiogenesis is regulated by potent anti-angiogenic factors such as thrombospondin, angiostatin, endostatin, vasostatin, and tumstatin. It seems that this balance is disturbed during tumor formation. Altered plasma levels of these inhibitor factors disrupt the balance [85]. Overexpression of RAS, succinate accumulation and loss of p53, and other growth factors initiate more and more HIF activity. Solid tumors are in hypoxic environments, which induce angiogenic factors such as VEGF, ANG1, IL8, osteopontin, and FGF.

Along with altering inhibitor factors and more vascularization activation, some gene loss of function adds to angiogenesis. PML is a tumor suppressor gene that regulates HIF1 translation, and its loss causes excessive HIF activation [86]. Infiltration of macrophages, which requires PLGF, also stimulates angiogenesis [76]. How macrophages initiate more angiogenesis has yet to be made clear. HIF activation deficiency does not alter vascularization in all tumors. Knocking down HIF activity in tumor tissue sometimes activates other factors for angiogenesis and bypasses the HIF path. Both IL8 and VEGF expression knockdown, on the other hand, seem to reduce tumor angiogenesis according to animal studies and might be a treatment target for solid tumors [86].

Predictions

Vascular mechanisms related to chronic diseases such as Alzheimer's disease, orogastric ulcerations, hair loss, age-related nephropathy, and osteoporosis will be discussed in the respective chapters. Finally, we will summarize the predicted near-future of improvements in the genes related to vascularization.

Atherosclerosis is a vastly complicated disease. Understanding the genetics of atherosclerosis in detail will be beneficial to distinguish pharmacological interventions. Recently gene therapies have been discussed for atherosclerosis prevention. PCSK9 is a primary target for new pharmaceutical trials. Monoclonal antibodies of this protein are being considered for hyperlipidemia treatment. There are investigations on new molecules such as alirocumab, evolocumab, and bococizumab. After the approach of a classical antiplatelet agent or statin therapy, this could be a major improvement [87]. Another idea about gene therapy for atherosclerosis is clustered regularly interspaced short palindromic repeat (CRISPR), which means modifying the gene or transplanting the modified coded tissue. Animal studies focus on that subject [88]. This method targets more than one gene. PCSK9, ApoB, and ApoC3 are the potential targets of new knock-out technics. HDL surface protein ApoA1 might be another target. ApoA1 is responsible for reverse cholesterol transport, acting as an anti-inflammatory and antioxidant. Animal data with ApoA1 modification shows decreased plaque volume and repressed inflammation [89]. Peroxisome proliferator-activated receptors (PPAR)-gamma is a regulator that facilitates cholesterol efflux. Animal data informs us that this molecule's overexpression stabilizes atherosclerotic plaques and knocking out PPAR rescues blood flow, but not diminishes plaque density [90]. Immunoreaction control genes are also targets for atherosclerosis treatment. This research started with MCP1, which reduces inflammatory cell infiltration [91]. The liver X receptors (LXR), LXRA, and LXRB, form a subfamily of the nuclear receptor superfamily and are key regulators of macrophage function, controlling transcriptional programs involved in lipid homeostasis and inflammation. LXRA also increases the expression of cholesterol efflux genes such as ABCA1 and ApoE. In addition that these receptors are involved in regulating cytokine production [92]. All chemokines involving the recruitment and migration of inflammatory cells and cytokines might also be treatment targets. In-stent restenosis and stent thrombosis may be developed after treatment methods of atherosclerosis, such as angioplasty and stent implantation. New gene therapies target these processes to prevent it from occurring and treat atherosclerosis. Local transferring of specific genes has been verified to be effective in inhibiting neointimal hyperplasia and no atherosclerosis. iNOS, VEGF, MCP1, TGFB1, tumor-derived protein tissue inhibitor of metalloproteinases-1 (TIMP1) are among these genes. Stents are being used to locally transferring genes. For example, the delivery of iNOS increases local NO and inhibits the adhesion of platelets and macrophages. VEGF delivery ensures the regeneration of endothelial cells. TIMP1 delivery inhibits matrix metalloproteinases, which promote the proliferation and migration of muscle cells and degrade the extra-cellular matrix [93]. Of course, transferring a single gene cannot achieve the preferred effect, but combining it with two or more might be a better solution. Another method for treating cardiovascular diseases is using modified endothelial progenitor cells. Recent studies suggest that properly selected and modified EPCs could be utilized either for stimulatory or inhibitory therapeutic purposes related to vasculogenesis. This method depends on transplanting progenitor cells cultured with specific molecules to ischemic tissue. Various growth factors such as FGF, VEGF, FL (fms-like tyrosine kinase 3 (FLT3) ligand), thrombopoietin, IL3 and 6, EPO, and stem cell factor have been selected for this process [94]. Recently, cell therapy for ischemic limb disease due to diabetes or atherosclerosis has been tried [95]. Since EPCs are known to migrate to areas of tumor vasculogenesis and angiogenesis selectively, these cells could be modified to deliver toxins, suicide genes, and drugs that interfere with tumor progression, vasculogenesis, and angiogenesis. For example, modified CD40L-expressing endothelial cells increased tumor cell apoptosis and augmented cytotoxicity toward tumor cells [96].

Under normal circumstances, the dominant way tumors obtain their vasculature is through angiogenesis. Vasculogenesis can be referred to as backup if angiogenesis is somehow inhibited. Recently, it has been shown that radiotherapy prevents the angiogenesis process of tumors [97]. Therefore, if vasculogenesis can be blocked too, solid tumors would become more fragile to radiation. It is observed that after radiation therapy, tumor tissue is invaded by macrophages. This invasion occurs thanks to SDF1 and HIF1 expression increase. After HIF inhibition in animal studies, this macrophage infiltration seems to be abolished [98]. Other studies suggest that HIF deficiency makes tumor tissue more sensitive to radiation but does not affect the growth of unirradiated tumors [99]. But today, HIF inhibition is an issue due to the lack of a specific inhibitor, and the HIF path includes many other molecular control. But another molecule could be selected downstream of the HIF pathway. SDF1 is one of these options. SDF levels also increase in irradiated tissue [100]. SDF1 functions as a chemoattractant for inflammatory cells and works through two receptors: CXCR4 and CXCR7. Clinical trial for plerixafor (a specific inhibitor of SDF1 and CXCR4 interaction) following irradiation therapy shows that tumor vasculature does not return [101]. HIF and SDF inhibition prevents myeloid cell migration in tumors and makes the tissue more sensitive to radiation. In addition, today, a series of angiogenesis inhibitors are being used for cancer treatment. Gefitinib is an EGFR inhibitor that blocks some of the proangiogenic factors. Bevacizumab is a monoclonal antibody of VEGF and sunitinib is the non-selective VEGF receptor blocker.

Bevacizumab is the first FDA-approved anti-angiogenic drug. Today more and more inhibitors are being approved for treatment. Axitinib is used for renal cell carcinoma treatment by inhibiting VEGFR1-3, c-KIT, and PDGFR [102]. Cabozantinib is used against thyroid medullary and renal cell carcinoma by inhibiting VEGFR, RET, and FLT3 [103]. Lenalidomide is used to treat both inflammatory disorders and multiple myeloma. It induces tumor cell apoptosis as well as angiogenesis inhibition. Lenvatinib mesylate treats thyroid cancer by inhibiting VEGFR1-3, FGFR, and PDGFR [104]. Pazopanib is another inhibitor of VEGFR, PDGFR, c-KIT, and FGFR [105]. Ramucirumab is a direct VEGFR2 antagonist, which leads to the inhibition of VEGF-mediated tumor angiogenesis [106]. Regorafenib shows anti-angiogenic activity due to its dual-targeted VEGFR2-TIE2 tyrosine kinase inhibition. It is used to treat advanced gastrointestinal carcinomas. Sorafenib treats renal cell, hepatocellular, and thyroid carcinoma by inhibiting VEGFR, PDGFR, and RAF kinases [107]. Sunitinib inhibits cellular signaling by targeting multiple receptor tyrosine kinases that include all receptors for a platelet-derived growth factor (PDGF-Rs) and vascular endothelial growth factor receptors (VEGFRs), which play a role in both tumor angiogenesis and tumor cell proliferation [108]. Vandetanib is another blocker of VEGFR2, EGFR, and RET tyrosine kinases and weakly inhibits VEGFR3 [109]. Aflibercept binds to circulating VEGFs and acts like a "VEGF trap." It thereby inhibits the activity of the vascular endothelial growth factor subtypes VEGF-A and VEGF-B, as well as to placental growth factor (PGF), inhibiting the growth of new blood vessels in the choriocapillaris or the tumor [110]. Bortezomib is a proteasome inhibitor that is being used for the treatment of multiple myeloma treatment nowadays [111]. Erlotinib, cetuximab, and vandetanib are developed as EGFR inhibitors. Lately, these drugs have also been found to inhibit the VEGF receptor [112]. These drugs are being used in clinics for treatment, but trials of new molecules are also underway. 2-Methoxyestradiol targets the tumor vasculature by inhibiting HIF1a and tubular formation. Everolimus, vatalanib, CCI-779, AZD2171, AMG706 are blockers of VEGFR. Neovastat, BMS-275291, and prinomastat are all matrix metalloproteinase inhibitors. Phosphomannopentaose sulfate stimulates the release of TFP1. Suramin is the non-selective blocker of EGFR, PDGFR, VEGF, and bFGF. These and more molecules are under phase studies.

Conclusion

Many diseases have genetic properties. For this reason, we are investigating more about genetics. For example, genetic diagnostic methods and therapies have recently become an undeniable part of cancer treatment. Increasing knowledge of genetic control of vascular development opens new paths for developing the most challenging medical treatments. New studies are rapidly increasing nowadays to understand unknown paths of this control.

References

[1] Risau, Werner; Flamme, Ingo (1995). Vasculogenesis. *Annual Review of Cell and Developmental Biology*, 11(1), 73–91. doi:10.1146/annurev.cb.11.110195.000445.

[2] Mitrani E, Gruenbaum Y, Shohat H, Ziv T. 1990. Fibroblast growth factor during mesoderm induction in the early chick embryo. *Development* 109:387-93.

[3] Dyer MA, Farrington SM, Mohn D, Munday JR, Baron MH. Indian hedgehog activates hematopoiesis and vasculogenesis and can respecify prospective neuroectodermal cell fate in the mouse embryo. *Development* 128: 1717-1730,2001.

[4] Kattman, S. J., Adler, E. D., Keller, G. M. (2007). Specification of multipotential cardiovascular progenitor cells during embryonic stem cell differentiation and embryonic development. *Trends in cardiovascular medicine*, 17(7), 240-246.

[5] Poole TJ, Finkelstein EB, Cox CM. The role of FGF and VEGF in angioblast induction and migration during vascular development. *Dev Dyn* 2001; 220:1-17.

[6] Papanayotou C, Collignon J. Activin/Nodal signalling before implantation: setting the stage for embryo patterning. *Philos Trans R Soc Lond B Biol Sci.* 2014;369 (1657):20130539. doi:10.1098/rstb.2013.0539.

[7] Abdulla, R. I., Blew, G. A., Holterman, M. J. (2004). Cardiovascular embryology. *Pediatric cardiology*, 25, 191-200.

[8] Jones CM, Dale L, Hogan BL, Wright CV, Smith JC. Bone morphogenetic protein-4 (BMP-4) acts during gastrula stages to cause ventralization of Xenopus embryos. *Development*. 1996 May 1;122(5):1545-54.

[9] Green JBA, New HV, Smith JC. 1992. Responses of embryonic Xenopus cells to activin and lGI are separated by multiple dose thresholds and correspond to distinct axes of the mesoderm. *Cell* 71:731-39.

[10] Johansson, BM, Wiles MV. 1995. Evidence for involvement of activin A and bone morphogenetic protein 4 in mammalian mesoderm and haematopoietic development. *Mol. Cell. Biol.* 15: 141-151.

[11] Winnier G, Blessing M, Labosky PA, Hogan BL. Bone morphogenetic protein-4 is required for mesoderm formation and patterning in the mouse. *Genes Dev* 1995; 9:2105-116.

[12] Dorey K, Amaya E. FGF signalling: diverse roles during early vertebrate embryogenesis. *Development*. 2010;137(22):3731-3742. doi:10.1242/dev.037689.

[13] Xu, RH, Ault, KT, Kim, J, Park, MJ, Hwang, YS, Peng, Y, Sredni, D. Hf, K. (1999) Opposite effects of FGF and BMP-4 on embryonic blood formation: roles of PV.1 and GATA-2. *Dev. Biol*. 208, 352–361.

[14] Standley, HJ, Zorn, AM. Gurdon, JB. (2001) eFGF and its mode of action in the community effect during Xenopus myogenesis. *Development* 128, 1347–1357.

[15] Harry V. Isaacs; Anne E. Deconinck; Mary E. Pownall (2007). FGF4 regulates blood and muscle specification in *Xenopus laevis*, *Biol Cell.* 99(3), 165–173. doi:10.1042/bc20060103.

[16] G. Breier, U. Albrecht, S. Sterrer, W. Risau; Expression of vascular endothelial growth factor during embryonic angiogenesis and endothelial cell differentiation. *Development* 1 February 1992; 114 (2): 521–532.

[17] Quinn, T. P., Peters, K. G., De Vries, C., Ferrara, N., Williams, L. T. Fetal liver kinase 1 is a receptor for vascular endothelial growth factor and is selectively expressed in vascular endothelium. *Proc. Nat. Acad. Sci.* 90: 7533-7537, 1993.

[18] Gerwins, P., Sköldenberg, E., Claesson-Welsh, L. (2000). Function of fibroblast growth factors and vascular endothelial growth factors and their receptors in angiogenesis. *Critical reviews in oncology/hematology*, 34(3), 185-194.

[19] Takashima S, Kitakaze M, Asakura M, Asanuma H, Sanada S, Tashiro F, Niwa H, Miyazaki JI, Hirota S, Kitamura Y, Kitsukawa T. Targeting of both mouse neuropilin-1 and neuropilin-2 genes severely impairs developmental yolk sac and embryonic angiogenesis. *Proceedings of the National Academy of Sciences*. 2002 Mar 19;99(6):3657-62.

[20] Breier G, Albrecht U, Sterrer S, Risau W. Expression of vascular endothelial growth factor during embryonic angiogenesis and endothelial cell differentiation. *Development*. 1992 Feb 1;114(2):521-32.

[21] Yamashita, J., Itoh, H., Hirashima, M., Ogawa, M., Nishikawa, S., Yurugi, T., Naito, M., Nakao, K., Nishikawa, S.-I. Flk1-positive cells derived from embryonic stem cells serve as vascular progenitors. *Nature* 408: 92-96, 2000.

[22] He, Y., Smith, S. K., Day, K. A., Clark, D. E., Licence, D. R., Charnock-Jones, D. S. Alternative splicing of vascular endothelial growth factor (VEGF)-R1 (FLT-1) pre-mRNA is important for the regulation of VEGF activity. *Molec. Endocr.* 13: 537-545, 1999.

[23] Nakazawa F, Nagai H, Shin M, Sheng G. Negative regulation of primitive hematopoiesis by the FGF signaling pathway. *Blood*. 2006 Nov 15;108(10):3335-43.

[24] Lai L, Bohnsack BL, Niederreither K, Hirschi KK. Retinoic acid regulates endothelial cell proliferation during vasculogenesis. *Development* 2003; 130:6465-74.

[25] Palis J, Malik J, Mcgrath KE, Kingsley PD. Primitive erythropoiesis in the mammalian embryo. *International Journal of Developmental Biology*. 2010 Jul 17;54(6-7):1011-8.

[26] Patan S, Tanda S, Roberge S, Jones RC, Jain RK, Munn LL. Vascular morphogenesis and remodeling in a human tumor xenograft. Blood vessel

formation and growth in the ovarian pedicle after ovariectomy. *Circ. Res.* 89:723-731, 200 I.

[27] Pober, JS. (2012) Just the FACS or stalking the elusive circulating endothelial progenitor cell. *Arterioscler Thromb Vasc Biol* 32: 837–838.

[28] Zengin, E, F. Chalajour, UM. Gehling, WD. Ito, H. Treede, H. Lauke, J. Weil, H. Reichenspurner, N. Kilic, S. Ergun (2006) Vascular wall resident progenitor cells: a source for postnatal vasculogenesis. *Development* 133: 1543–1551.

[29] Kurz, H, Burri, PH, Djonov, VG. (2003). Angiogenesis and Vascular Remodeling by Intussusception: From Form to Function. *Physiology*, 18(2), 65–70. doi:10. 1152/nips.01417.2002.

[30] Dumont OJ, Fong G-H, Puri MC, Gradwohl G, Alitalo K, Breitman ML. Vascularization ofthe mouse embryo: A study offlk-I, tek, tie, and vascular endothelial growth factor expression during development. *Dev. Dyn.* 203: 80-92, 1995.

[31] Patan S. TIEl and TIE2 receptor tyrosine kinases inversely regulate embryonic angiogenesis by the mechanism of intussusceptive microvascular growth. *Microvasc. Res.* 56: 1-21, 1998.

[32] Witzenbichler B, Maisonpierre PC, Jones P, Yancopoulos GD, Isner JM. Chemotactic properties of angiopoietin-I and -2, ligands for the endothelial-specific receptor tyrosine kinase Tie2. *J. BioI. Chern.* 273: 18514-18521, 1998.

[33] Asahara T, Chen D, Takahashi T, Fujikawa K, Kearney M, Magner M, Yancopoulos GD, Isner JM. Tie2 receptor ligands, angiopoietin-I and angiopoietin-2, modulate VEGF-induced postnatal neovascularization. *Circ. Res.* 83: 233-240, 1998.

[34] Sato TN, Tozawa Y, Deutsch U, Wolburg-Buchholz K, Fujiwara Y, Gendron-Maguire M, Gridley T, Wolburg H, Risau W, Quin Y. Distinct roles ofthe receptor tyrosine kinases TIEl and TlE2 in blood vessel formation. *Nature* 376: 70-74, 1995.

[35] Adams RH, Wilkinson GA, Weiss C, Die1laF, Gale NW, Deutsch U, Risau W, Klein R. Roles of ephrin-B ligands and EphB receptors in cardiovascular development: Demarcation of arterial/venous domains, vascular morphogenesis, and sprouting angiogenesis. *Genes Dev.* 3: 295-306, 1999.

[36] Carmeliet P (2003). *Angiogenesis in health and disease.*, 9(6), 653–660. doi:10.1038/nm0603-653.

[37] Garcia-Porrero JA, Godin IE, Dieterlen-Lievre F. Potential intraembryonic hemogenic sites at pre-liver stages in the mouse. *Anat Embryol* 1995; 192:425-35.

[38] Wang L, Li L, Shojaei F, Levac K, Cerdan C, Menendez P, Martin T, Rouleau A, Bhatia M. Endothelial and hematopoietic cell fate of human embryonic stem cells originates from primitive endothelium with hemangioblastic properties. *Immunity.* 2004 Jul 1;21(1):31-41.

[39] Mikkola, H., Fujiwara, Y., Schlaeger, T., Traver, D., Orkin, S. (2002). Expression of CD41 marks the initiation of definitive hematopoiesis in the mouse embryo. *Blood* doi 10.1182/blood-2002-06-1699.

[40] Tam PPL, Behringer RR. Mouse gastrulation: the formation of a mammalian body plan. *Mech Dev* 1997; 68:3-25.

[41] Shalaby F, Rossant J, Yamaguchi TP, Gertsenstein M, Wu XF, Breitman ML, Schuh AC. Failure of blood-island formation and vasculogenesis in Flk-1-deficient mice. *Nature.* 1995 Jul 6;376(6535):62-6.

[42] Damert, A., Miquerol, L., Gertsenstein, M., Risau, W., Nagy, A. Insufficient VEGFA activity in yolk sac endoderm compromises haematopoietic and endothelial differentiation. *Development* 2002; 129:1881-92.

[43] Shalaby F, Ho J, Stanford WL, Fischer KD, Schuh AC, Schwartz L, Bernstein A, Rossant J. A requirement for Flk1 in primitive and definitive hematopoiesis and vasculogenesis. *Cell.* 1997 Jun 13;89(6):981-90.

[44] Robertson SM, Kennedy M, Shannon JM, Keller G. A transitional stage in the commitment of mesoderm to hematopoiesis requiring the transcription factor SCL/Tal-1. *Development* 2000; 127:2447-59.

[45] Fujiwara Y, Browne CP, Cunniff K, Goff SC, Orkin SH. Arrested development of embryonic red cell precursors in mouse embryos lacking transcription factor GATA-1. *Proceedings of the National Academy of Sciences.* 1996 Oct 29;93(22): 12355-8.

[46] Tsai FY, Keller G, Kuo FC, Weiss M, Chen J, Rosenblatt M, Alt FW, Orkin SH. An early haematopoietic defect in mice lacking the transcription factor GATA-2. *Nature.* 1994 Sep 15;371(6494):221-6.

[47] Okuda T, Van Deursen J, Hiebert SW, Grosveld G, Downing JR. AML1, the target of multiple chromosomal translocations in human leukemia, is essential for normal fetal liver hematopoiesis. *Cell.* 1996 Jan 26;84(2):321-30.

[48] North TE, De Bruijn MF, Stacy T, Talebian L, Lind E, Robin C, Binder M, Dzierzak E, Speck NA. Runx1 expression marks long-term repopulating hematopoietic stem cells in the midgestation mouse embryo. *Immunity.* 2002 May 1;16(5):661-72.

[49] Yamada Y, Pannell R, Forster A, Rabbitts TH. The oncogenic LIM-only transcription factor Lmo2 regulates angiogenesis but not vasculogenesis in mice. *Proc Natl Acad Sci USA* 2000; 97:320-4.

[50] Palis, J., Chan, R., Koniski, A., Patel, R., Starr, M., Yoder, M. (2001). Spatial and temporal emergence of high proliferative potential hematopoietic precursors during murine embryogenesis. *Proc. Natl. Acad. Sci. USA* 98, 4528-4533.

[51] Ferkowicz, M. J. (2003). CD41 expression defines the onset of primitive and definitive hematopoiesis in the murine embryo. *Development*, 130(18), 4393–4403. doi:10.1242/dev.00632.

[52] Gekas C, Graf T. CD41 expression marks myeloid-biased adult hematopoietic stem cells and increases with age. *Blood.* 2013;121(22):4463-4472. doi:10.1182/blood-2012-09-457929.

[53] Herrmann F, Groß A, Zhou D, Kestler HA, Kühl M. A boolean model of the cardiac gene regulatory network determining first and second heart field identity. *PLoS One*. 2012;7(10):e46798. doi:10.1371/journal.pone.0046798.

[54] Reamon-Buettner SM, Ciribilli Y, Traverso I, Kuhls B, Inga A, Borlak J. A functional genetic study identifies HAND1 mutations in septation defects of the human heart. *Human molecular genetics.* 2009 Oct 1;18(19):3567-78.

[55] Russell MW, Kemp P, Wang L, Brody LC, Izumo S. Molecular cloning of the human HAND2 gene. *Biochimica et Biophysica Acta (BBA)-Gene Structure and Expression*. 1998 Dec 22;1443(3):393-9.

[56] Kitajima S, Takagi A, Inoue T, Saga Y (2000) MesP1 and MesP2 are essential for the development of cardiac mesoderm. *Development* 127: 3215–3226.

[57] Lescroart, F., Wang, X., Lin, X., Swedlund, B., Gargouri, S., Sanchez-Danes, A., Moignard, V., Dubois, C., Paulissen, C., Kinston, S., Gottgens, B., Blanpain, C. Defining the earliest step of cardiovascular lineage segregation by single-cell RNA-seq. *Science* 359: 1177-181, 2018.

[58] Buckingham M, Meilhac S, Zaffran S. Building the mammalian heart from two sources of myocardial cells. *Nat Rev Genet.* 2005;6(11):826-835. doi:10.1038/nrg1710.

[59] Xavier-Neto J, Neville CM, Shapiro MD, Houghton L, Wang GF, Nikovits W, Stockdale FE, Rosenthal N. A retinoic acid-inducible transgenic marker of sino-atrial development in the mouse heart. *Development*. 1999 Jun 19;126(12):2677-87.

[60] Wessels A, Phelps A, Trusk TC, Davis DL, Edwards AV, Burch JB, Juraszek AL. Mouse models for cardiac conduction system development. In *Development of the Cardiac Conduction System: Novartis Foundation Symposium 250*. 2003 Jun 20 (Vol. 250, pp. 44-67). Chichester, UK: John Wiley & Sons, Ltd.

[61] Liberatore CM, Searcy-Schrick RD, Yutzey KE. Ventricular expression of tbx5 inhibits normal heart chamber development. *Dev Biol* 223: 169–180, 2000.

[62] Bruneau BG, Nemer G, Schmitt JP, Charron F, Robitaille L, Caron S, Conner DA, Gessler M, Nemer M, Seidman CE, Seidman JG. A murine model of Holt-Oram syndrome definesroles of the T-box transcription factor Tbx5 in cardiogenesis anddisease. *Cell 106*: 709–721, 2001.

[63] Xu H, Morishima M, Wylie JN, Schwartz RJ, Bruneau BG, Lindsay EA, Baldini A. Tbx1 has a dual role in the morphogenesis of the cardiac outflow tract. *Development*. 2004;131(13):3217-3227. doi:10.1242/dev.01174.

[64] Cai CL, Liang X, Shi Y, Chu PH, Pfaff SL, Chen J, Evans S. Isl1 identifies a cardiac progenitor population that proliferates prior to differentiation and contributes a majority of cells to the heart. *Developmental cell*. 2003 Dec 1;5(6):877-89.

[65] Guo Y, Dorn T, Kühl SJ, Linnemann A, Rothe M, Pfister AS, Vainio S, Laugwitz KL, Moretti A, Kühl M. The Wnt inhibitor Dkk1 is required for maintaining the normal cardiac differentiation program in *Xenopus laevis*. *Developmental biology*. 2019 May 1;449(1):1-3.

[66] Kitajima, S., Takagi, A., Inoue, T., Saga, Y. MesP1 and MesP2 are essential for the development of cardiac mesoderm. *Development* 127, 3215–3226 (2003).

[67] Ausprunk D, Folkman J. Migration and proliferation of endothelial cells in preformed and newly formed blood vessels during tumor angiogenesis. *Microvasc. Res*. 14: 53-65, 1977.

[68] Kelly BD, Hackett SF, Hirota K, Oshima Y, Cai Z, BergDixon S, Rowan A, Yan Z, Campochiaro PA, Semenza GL. 2003. Cell type-specific regulation of angiogenic growth factor gene expression and induction of angiogenesis in

nonischemic tissue by a constitutively active form of hypoxia-inducible factor 1. *Circ Res* 93:1074–1081.

[69] Stoeltzing O, McCarty MF, Wey JS, Fan F, Liu W, Belcheva A, Bucana CD, Semenza GL, Ellis LM. 2004. Role of hypoxia-inducible factor 1a in gastric cancer cell growth, angiogenesis, and vessel maturation. *J Natl Cancer Inst* 96:946–956.

[70] Martin P, Leibovich SJ (2005) Inflammatory cells during wound repair: the good, the bad and the ugly. *Trends Cell Biol* 15(11):599–607.

[71] Jin DK, Shido K, Kopp HG, Petit I, Shmelkov SV, Young LM, Hooper AT, Amano H, Avecilla ST, Heissig B, Hattori K, Zhang F, Hicklin DJ, Wu Y, Zhu Z, Dunn A, Salari H, Werb Z, Hackett NR, Crystal RG, Lyden D, Rafii S. 2006. Cytokine-mediated deployment of SDF-1 induces revascularization through recruitment of CXCR4þ hemangiocytes. *Nat Med* 12:557–567.

[72] Wang GL, Jiang BH, Rue EA, Semenza GL. 1995. Hypoxiainducible factor 1 is a basic-helix-loop-helix-PAS heterodimer regulated by cellular O2 tension. *Proc Natl Acad Sci USA* 92:5510–5514.

[73] Shyu KG, Wang MT, Wang BW, Chang CC, Leu JG, Kuan P, Chang H. Intramyocardial injection of naked DNA encoding HIF-1α/VP16 hybrid to enhance angiogenesis in an acute myocardial infarction model in the rat. *Cardiovascular research*. 2002 Jun 1;54(3):576-83.

[74] Davidson JD, Mustoe TA (2001) Oxygen in wound healing: more than a nutrient. *Wound Repair Regen* 9(3):175–177.

[75] Isner JM (1999) Cancer and atherosclerosis: the broad mandate of angiogenesis. *Circulation* 99(13):1653–1655

[76] Mani A, Radhakrishnan J, Wang HE, Mani A, Mani MA, Nelson-Williams C, Carew KS, Mane S, Najmabadi H, Wu D, Lifton RP. LRP6 mutation in a family with early coronary disease and metabolic risk factors. *Science*. 2007 Mar 2;315(5816):1278-82.

[77] Chang KH, Chan-Ling T, McFarland EL, Afzal A, Pan H, Baxter LC, Shaw LC, Caballero S, Sengupta N, Calzi SL, Sullivan SM. IGF binding protein-3 regulates hematopoietic stem cell and endothelial precursor cell function during vascular development. *Proceedings of the National Academy of Sciences*. 2007 Jun 19;104(25):10595-600.

[78] Ma, X, Bacci, S, Mlynarski, W, Gottardo, L, Soccio, T, Menzaghi, C, Iori, E, Lager, RA, Shroff, AR, Gervino, EV, Nesto, RW, Johnstone, MT, Abumrad, NA, Avogaro, A, Trischitta, V, Doria, A. A common haplotype at the CD36 locus is associated with high free fatty acid levels and increased cardiovascular risk in Caucasians. *Hum. Molec. Genet.* 13: 2197-2205, 2004. Note: Erratum: Hum. Molec. Genet. 13: 3973 only, 2005.

[79] Weng, L., Kavaslar, N., Ustaszewska, A., Doelle, H., Schackwitz, W., Hebert, S., Cohen, J. C., McPherson, R., Pennacchio, L. A. Lack of MEF2A mutations in coronary artery disease. *J. Clin. Invest.* 115: 1016-1020, 2005.

[80] Cao G, Xuan X, Zhang R, Hu J, Dong H. Gene Therapy for Cardiovascular Disease: Basic Research and Clinical Prospects. *Front Cardiovasc Med.* 2021;8:760140. Published 2021 Nov 5. doi:10.3389/fcvm.2021.760140.

[81] Lima e Silva R, Shen J, Hackett SF, Kachi S, Akiyama H, Kiuchi K, Yokoi K, Hatara MC, Lauer T, Aslam S, Gong YY. The SDF-1/CXCR4 ligand/receptor pair is an important contributor to several types of ocular neovascularization. *The FASEB Journal*. 2007 Oct;21(12):3219-3230.

[82] Peters CL, Morris CJ, Mapp PI, Blake DR, Lewis CE, Winrow VR. The transcription factors hypoxia-inducible factor 1α and Ets-1 colocalize in the hypoxic synovium of inflamed joints in adjuvant-induced arthritis. *Arthritis & Rheumatism: Official Journal of the American College of Rheumatology*. 2004 Jan;50(1):291-296.

[83] Dudek AZ, Mahaseth H (2005) Circulating angiogenic cytokines in patients with advanced non-small cell lung cancer: correlation with treatment response and survival. *Cancer Invest* 23(3):193–200.

[84] Guo-Hua F (2008). *Mechanisms of adaptive angiogenesis to tissue hypoxia.,* 11(2), 121–140. doi:10.1007/s10456-008-9107-3.

[85] Bernardi R, Guernah I, Jin D, Grisendi S, Alimonti A, Teruya-Feldstein J, Cordon-Cardo C, Celeste Simon M, Rafii S, Pandolfi PP. PML inhibits HIF-1α translation and neoangiogenesis through repression of mTOR. *Nature*. 2006 Aug 17;442(7104):779-85.

[86] Lusis AJ, Mar R, Pajukanta P. Genetics of atherosclerosis. *Annu. Rev. Genomics Hum. Genet.*. 2004 Sep 22;5:189-218.

[87] Thorne, R. G., Nicholson, C. (2006). In vivo diffusion analysis with quantum dots and dextrans predicts the width of brain extracellular space. *Proceedings of the National Academy of Sciences*, 103(14), 5567-5572.

[88] Wacker BK, Dronadula N, Zhang J, Dichek DA. Local vascular gene therapy with apolipoprotein A-I. to promote regression of atherosclerosis. *Arterioscler Thromb Vasc Biol.* (2017) 37:316–27.

[89] Theurl M, Schgoer W, Albrecht-Schgoer K, Lener D, Wolf D, Wolf M, Demetz E, Tymoszuk P, Tancevski I, Fischer-Colbrie R, Franz WM. Secretoneurin gene therapy improves hind limb and cardiac ischaemia in Apo E−/− mice without influencing systemic atherosclerosis. *Cardiovascular research*. 2015 Jan 1;105(1):96-106.

[90] Inoue, S, Egashira, K., Ni, W., Kitamoto, S., Usui, M., Otani, K., Takeshita, A. (2002). Anti-monocyte chemoattractant protein-1 gene therapy limits progression and destabilization of established atherosclerosis in apolipoprotein E–knockout mice. *Circulation*, 106(21), 2700-2706.

[91] Li, G., Biju, K. C., Xu, X., Zhou, Q., Chen, C., Valente, A. J., Li, S. (2011). Macrophage LXRα gene therapy ameliorates atherosclerosis as well as hypertriglyceridemia in LDLR−/− mice. *Gene therapy*, 18(8), 835-841.

[92] Correa, G. A. R., Zacchigna, S., Arsic, N., Zentilin, L., Salvi, A., Sinagra, G., Giacca, M. (2004). Potent inhibition of arterial intimal hyperplasia by TIMP1 gene transfer using AAV vectors. *Molecular Therapy*, 9(6), 876-884.

[93] Sukmawati, D, Tanaka R. (2015) Introduction to next generation of endothelial progenitor cell therapy: a promise in vascular medicine. *Am J Transl Res* 7: 411–421.

[94] Purwanti, Y. I., Chen, C., Lam, D. H., Wu, C., Zeng, J., Fan, W., Wang, S. (2014). Antitumor effects of CD40 ligand-expressing endothelial progenitor cells derived from human induced pluripotent stem cells in a metastatic breast cancer model. *Stem cells translational medicine*, 3(8), 923-935.

[95] Masuda, H., Iwasaki, H., Kawamoto, A., Akimaru, H., Ishikawa, M., Ii, M., Asahara, T. (2012). Development of serum-free quality and quantity control culture of colony-forming endothelial progenitor cell for vasculogenesis. *Stem cells translational medicine*, 1(2), 160-171.

[96] Ahn GO, Brown JM. Matrix metalloproteinase-9 is required for tumor vasculogenesis but not for angiogenesis: role of bone marrow-derived myelomonocytic cells. *Cancer Cell* 2008; 13: 193–205.

[97] Imaizumi, N., Monnier, Y., Hegi, M., Mirimanoff, R. O., Rüegg, C. (2010). Radiotherapy suppresses angiogenesis in mice through TGF-βRI/ALK5-dependent inhibition of endothelial cell sprouting. *PloS one*, 5(6), e11084.

[98] Chau NM, Rogers P, Aherne W, Carroll V, Collins I, McDonald E, Workman P, Ashcroft M. Identification of novel small molecule inhibitors of hypoxia-inducible factor-1 that differentially block hypoxia-inducible factor-1 activity and hypoxia-inducible factor-1α induction in response to hypoxic stress and growth factors. *Cancer Research*. 2005 Jun 1;65(11):4918-4928.

[99] Kozin SV, Kamoun WS, Huang Y, Dawson MR, Jain RK, Duda DG. Recruitment of myeloid but not endothelial precursor cells facilitates tumor regrowth after local irradiation. *Cancer Res* 2010; 70: 5679–85.

[100] Brown JM. Vasculogenesis: a crucial player in the resistance of solid tumours to radiotherapy. *Br J Radiol*. 2014;87(1035):20130686. doi:10.1259/bjr.20130686.

[101] DiPersio, J. F., Uy, G. L., Yasothan, U., Kirkpatrick, P. (2009). Plerixafor. *Nature reviews Drug discovery*, 8(2).

[102] Escudier B, Gore M (2011). "Axitinib for the management of metastatic renal cell carcinoma." *Drugs in R&D*. 11 (2): 113–26.

[103] Yakes, F. M., Chen, J., Tan, J., Yamaguchi, K., Shi, Y., Yu, P., Joly, A. H. (2011). Cabozantinib (XL184), a novel MET and VEGFR2 inhibitor, simultaneously suppresses metastasis, angiogenesis, and tumor growth. *Molecular cancer therapeutics*, 10(12), 2298-2308.

[104] Tohyama, O., Matsui, J., Kodama, K., Hata-Sugi, N., Kimura, T., Okamoto, K., Funahashi, Y. (2014). Antitumor activity of lenvatinib (e7080): an angiogenesis inhibitor that targets multiple receptor tyrosine kinases in preclinical human thyroid cancer models. *Journal of thyroid research*, 2014.

[105] Pick, AM; Nystrom, KK (2012). "Pazopanib for the treatment of metastatic renal cell carcinoma." *Clinical Therapeutics*. 34 (3): 511–520.

[106] Arrieta, O., Zatarain-Barrón, Z. L., Cardona, A. F., Carmona, A., Lopez-Mejia, M. (2017). Ramucirumab in the treatment of non-small cell lung cancer. *Expert Opinion on Drug Safety*, 16(5), 637-644.

[107] Wilhelm SM, Adnane L, Newell P, Villanueva A, Llovet JM, Lynch M (2008). "Preclinical overview of sorafenib, a multikinase inhibitor that targets both Raf and VEGF and PDGF receptor tyrosine kinase signaling." *Mol Cancer Ther*. 7 (10): 3129–40.

[108] " Goodman, VL, Rock, EP, Dagher, R, Ramchandani, RP, Abraham, S, Gobburu, JV, Pazdur, R. (2007). Approval summary: sunitinib for the treatment of imatinib refractory or intolerant gastrointestinal stromal tumors and advanced renal cell carcinoma. *Clinical Cancer Research*, 13(5), 1367-1373.

[109] Carlomagno, F, Vitagliano, D, Guida, T, Ciardiello, F, Tortora, G, Vecchio, G, Ryan, AJ, Fontanini, G, Fusco, A, Santoro, M (2002). "ZD6474, an orally available inhibitor of KDR tyrosine kinase activity, efficiently blocks oncogenic RET kinases." *Cancer Research*. 62 (24): 7284–90.

[110] Ciombor, KK, Berlin, J, Chan, E. (2013). Aflibercept and Its Role in the Treatment of Colorectal Cancer. *Clinical Cancer Research*, 19(8), 1920-1925.

[111] Bonvini, P, Zorzi, E, Basso, G, Rosolen, A. (2007). Bortezomib-mediated 26S proteasome inhibition causes cell-cycle arrest and induces apoptosis in CD-30+ anaplastic large cell lymphoma. *Leukemia*, 21(4), 838-842.

[112] Folkman, J. (2007). Angiogenesis: an organizing principle for drug discovery?. *Nature reviews Drug discovery*, 6(4), 273-286.

Chapter 4

Vascularization and Infection

Oguz Evlice[1,*], MD
Department of Infectious Diseases and Clinical Microbiology,
Kutahya University of Health Sciences School of Medicine, Kutahya, Turkey

Abstract

The vascular system carries the main requirements, such as blood and oxygen, to the body. There are five distinct components of the circulatory system: arteries and arterioles (arterial system), veins and venules (venous system), and capillaries (microvascular system) that link arterioles and venules. Blood vessels play a critical role in homeostasis and contribute to disease pathophysiology in almost every organ system. Therefore, an understanding of vascular biology provides insight into most diseases. Endothelial cells are critical in the systemic response to infection and organ dysfunction. The pathophysiology of coagulation disorders due to endothelial dysfunction and disseminated intravascular coagulation is poorly understood. The development of therapies targeting endothelial cells may help reduce mortality due to infectious diseases.

Keywords: sepsis, COVID-19, endothelial dysfunction, microvascular thrombosis, endothelial cells

Introduction

Blood vessels play a crucial role in homeostasis and contribute to disease pathophysiology in almost every organ system. Therefore, an understanding

* Corresponding Author's Email: oguzevlice@hotmail.com.

In: Vascularization and Its Role in Medicine and Tissue Engineering
Editors: Emre Bulbul and Murat Oguz Ozilhan
ISBN: 979-8-89113-041-8

of vascular biology provides insight into most diseases. Veins and arteries typically form a three-layered structure. The inner layer consists of a single layer of endothelium. The middle layer consists of smooth muscle cells. The outer layer consists of a loose extracellular matrix containing rare fibroblasts, mast cells, and nerve endings. Large arteries have a vascular system called the vasa vasorum, extending to the tunica media's outer parts [1]. The vascular endothelium has many functions. The most prominent role of the endothelium is to provide a surface between the tissues and the blood compartment. Thus, it selectively regulates the entry of cells and molecules into the tissues. Unfortunately, endothelial cells' selective permeable barrier function is impaired in most vascular diseases, including atherosclerosis and hypertension.

The endothelium also regulates local blood flow and vascular tonus: Nitric oxide (NO) and prostacyclin are produced by endothelial cells and exert vasodilatory effects. In pathological conditions, the overproduction of reactive oxygen compounds produced by endothelial cells and smooth muscle cells creates local oxidative stress and inactivates NO. The endothelial layer is also essential to the host's defence against infections. Intact endothelium is resistant to contact with leukocytes in the blood. However, when activated by bacterial products such as endotoxin or cytokines released during infection or injury, they exhibit leukocyte adhesion molecules to which different classes of leukocytes can bind. When activated by bacterial endotoxin or cytokines, endothelial cells can produce high amounts of plasminogen activator inhibitor-I, a significant fibrinolysis inhibitor. Thus, endothelial cells may cause local thrombus accumulation in pathologic conditions instead of fighting the thrombus. Inflammatory stimuli also stimulate the release of procoagulant tissue factor, which contributes to disseminated intravascular coagulation in sepsis. Tissue vascularisation can be impaired in many infectious diseases. Several infectious diseases can be mentioned as an example [2, 3].

Sepsis

Sepsis is organ dysfunction resulting from the host's dysregulated immunological response to infection. Sepsis remains a disease with a high mortality rate despite developing treatment methods. The pathophysiology of sepsis has been investigated in recent years. Although it has been essentially clarified, many unexplained situations still exist. Although there are some scoring systems for the detection of organ dysfunction, SOFA (Sequential/

Sepsis-related Organ Failure Assessment) is a well-known simple scoring system. Although not as powerful as SOFA, quick SOFA (qSOFA) can be applied easily in identifying adult patients with suspected infections. qSOFA score includes 1 point for each of the three criteria: respiratory rate ≥ 22 breaths/min, altered mental status, or systolic blood pressure (SBP) ≤ 100 mm Hg. A qSOFA score ≥ 2 is suggestive of sepsis [4].

The vascular endothelium regulates many physiological processes, and its dysfunction causes many diseases. Vascular endothelium has numerous physiological functions. It shows anticoagulant and antiadhesive activity, regulates vasomotor tonus and vascular hemostasis. Endothelial dysfunction has been explained by several pathophysiological mechanisms, such as oxidative stress and inflammation [5].

Endothelial barrier function is impaired during septic shock. The lipopolysaccharide layer in gram-negative bacteria and cytokines such as tumour necrosis factor (TNF)-alpha is involved in endothelial dysfunction. As a result, oedema occurs in vital organs such as the lung, kidney, or brain due to fluid passage into the extravascular space. In addition, there is increasing evidence that cell death secondary to apoptosis plays a role in the pathogenesis of septic shock. In vitro studies have demonstrated apoptosis-induced cell death induced by sepsis-related factors such as TNF-alpha or lipopolysaccharide [6, 7].

Free oxygen radicals are released secondary to sepsis-related inflammation and hypoxia. The resulting free oxygen radicals contribute to endothelial and tissue damage in septic shock. NO is generally secreted from the endothelium and is essential in maintaining vascular hemostasis. Overproduction of NO in sepsis contributes to hypotension and cardiac depression in septic shock [8].

Almost all the mediators involved in sepsis are effective on the vessels. Endotoxin, TNF-α, IL-1, platelet-activating factor, leukotrienes, and thromboxane A2 increase endothelium permeability. In addition, the activation of the complement cascade also causes endothelial damage. Activation of complement directly affects vessel permeability or indirectly by activating neutrophils. In addition, during degranulation, oxygen radicals released from neutrophils and lysosomal enzymes are released. It increases endothelial permeability. Increased vascular permeability and endothelial damage facilitate the formation of microthrombi. According to the extent of endothelial injury, organ failure occurs. The most common organ failure in sepsis; is lung, kidney, liver, and heart failure.

The coagulation system varies from mild laboratory abnormalities to DIC. One of the changes in the coagulation system in the direction of pro-coagulation is tissue factor-mediated thrombin generation. Tissue factor is secreted by endothelial cells or mononuclear cells. Endothelial dysfunction is a predictor of mortality in sepsis. Duffy et al., demonstrated that impaired endothelium-dependent vasodilation assessed by pulse wave analysis is associated with mortality in critical illness [9]. Endothelial cells are essential in the systemic response to infection and organ dysfunction. The pathophysiology of coagulation disorders due to endothelial dysfunction and disseminated intravascular coagulation is poorly understood. The development of therapies targeting endothelial cells may help reduce sepsis-related mortality [10, 11].

COVID-19

Severe acute respiratory syndrome coronavirus 2 (SARS-COV-2) is an RNA virus that caused the pandemic called coronavirus disease-19 (COVID-19). While the disease is asymptomatic and mild, it can be severe and critical, especially in elderly patients with comorbidities. The most common clinical symptoms include fever, cough, dyspnea, sore throat, headache, fatigue, and myalgia [12]. In the course of the disease, systemic involvement, such as acute kidney injury, coagulation disorders, myocarditis, and pulmonary embolism, occur along with pneumonia. The predominance of systemic findings suggests vascular involvement [13, 14].

COVID-19-Associated Coagulopathy

Coagulopathy and thromboembolic events are common, especially in severe COVID-19. Therefore, anticoagulant prophylaxis is recommended in hospitalised patients with challenging clinical courses. Despite this, complications such as deep vein thrombosis and pulmonary embolism may occur in up to 30% of critically ill patients.

Proinflammatory cytokines secreted by macrophages in the lung cause thrombocytosis and hyperfibrinogenemia. This increase explains the coagulopathy in COVID-19. Proinflammatory cytokines are released similarly in many severe infections. However, there are some differences with COVID-19. For example, thrombocytopenia and prolonged prothrombin time are common in bacterial sepsis but not in COVID-19. In COVID-19, fibrinogen and D-dimer increase is more common [15, 16].

Endothelial dysfunction plays an essential role in the pathophysiology of viral infections. Endothelial dysfunction triggers coagulation disorders, especially in severe viral infections. The virus's direct effect on the endothelium or endothelial activation due to dysregulated immunologic response causes vascular leakage. Vascular leakage plays a critical role in endothelial dysfunction. During COVID-19, vascular inflammation causes endothelial damage with infiltration of mononuclear and lymphocyte cells. The endothelium plays an essential role in regulating vascular tone by synthesising vasodilators such as nitric oxide (NO) and prostaglandins and various vasoactive substances such as endothelium-dependent endothelin and angiotensin II [17].

Prophylactic anticoagulant therapy is recommended in patients with severe clinical course unless contraindicated. In a retrospective observational study, anticoagulant therapy was shown to reduce mortality (reduced risk of mortality: adjusted hazard ratio of 0.86 per day) [18, 19].

Microthrombosis in COVID-19

Microvascular thrombosis can occur in many infectious diseases, such as malaria and sepsis. It plays an essential role in multiple organ failures and mortality. In COVID-19, endothelial damage occurs through direct and indirect mechanisms. Cytokines, complement activation, activated platelets, and immune cells play a role in indirect damage. With the development of inactivated and mRNA vaccines, the impact of the COVID-19 pandemic is decreasing daily. However, endothelium-targeting therapies must be developed, especially in patients with a severe course. Microthrombosis, coagulopathy, and endothelial damage due to direct and indirect effects of the virus play an essential role in the pathophysiology of COVID-19. The development of targeted therapies will guide the treatment of not only COVID-19 but also many other viral and bacterial infections [20].

Endothelial Dysfunction in COVID-19

Vascular endothelium consists of a single layer of endothelial cells. It is located in the inner layer of arteries, veins, and capillaries. The endothelium also plays a critical role in maintaining vascular tone by secreting vasodilator and vasoconstrictor substances. It also maintains vascular hemostasis through NO synthesis. Endothelial dysfunction triggers coagulation disorders, especially in many viral infections. In our previous SARS experience, there were findings suggestive of endothelial dysfunction. The main target of the SARS-COV virus is lung and intestinal tissue, where angiotensin-converting enzyme 2 (ACE2) receptors are widely expressed [21, 22]. In addition, postmortem evaluation of SARS patients showed vasculitis and endothelial cell inflammation [23].

Diabetic Foot Infection

Foot ulcers affect one in ten patients with diabetes during their lifetime. These patients are at high risk of lower limb amputation, and the leading cause is a peripheral arterial disease. While minor debridement is sufficient in mild disease, major amputation may be required for severe disease. If there is the adequate blood supply to the infected foot, small vessel disease, and gangrenous fingers, debridement, and minor amputation may be sufficient in treatment. Primary amputation is preferred in wet gangrene, life-threatening sepsis, and in cases where revascularisation is not possible with extensive tissue necrosis [24].

Diabetic foot infection (DFI) can be prevented by providing foot care and controlling diabetes. In many cases, severe consequences can be avoided by early detection and treatment of a wound. There are many causes for developing DFI, but the leading cause is the combined effect of diabetes-related vascular disease and neuropathy [25].

Diabetic macroangiopathy and microangiopathy cause circulatory disturbances at the capillary level. Neuropathy and hyperglycemia particularly impair leukocyte diapedesis, chemotaxis, phagocytosis, and intracellular lysis. Additionally, they, coupled with impaired collagen metabolism, complicate the infection and wound healing.

In prolonged hyperglycemia, glucose nonenzymatically binds to proteins and triggers a series of reactions leading to the formation of so-called advanced glycosylation end products (AGE). These products bind to macrophages and cause low-level inflammation due to the release of many cytokines, especially TNF-α, and an increase in reactive oxygen species. In DFI wounds, this leads to apoptosis of fibroblasts and endothelial cells due to mitochondrial damage.

High blood glucose levels directly affect endothelial cells and vascular smooth muscle cells. In addition, hyperglycemia increases oxidative stress, leading to vascular complications [26]. Multiple factors contribute to the development of DFI. There is growing evidence that the most important mechanism is endothelial damage. Hyperglycemia causes oxidative stress in endothelial cells through pathways such as increased vascular permeability and decreased NO utilisation. Therefore, treatment options targeting the endothelium should be developed to treat DFI. An in vitro study showed that high blood glucose levels affect endothelial cells via the PKCβ-p66shc pathway [27]. Endothelial dysfunction is also thought to impair wound healing in DFI [28].

Revascularisation

Peripheral arterial disease (PAD) is observed in more than half of patients with diabetic foot ulcers. In the presence of DFI, vascular evaluation should be performed in every case possible. If a significant arterial insufficiency is present in a patient with DFI wounds, it should be recognised early and treated interventionally. Atherosclerotic arterial problems in diabetic patients are more distally located and are more likely to be occlusions than stenoses and involve multiple segments. In non-diabetic PAD, collateral development occurs against occlusion, whereas in diabetic patients, there are defects in the collateralization system. PAD in patients with diabetes typically affects the vessels between the knee and ankle. Therefore, its treatment is critical in wound healing if the PAD is present.

If PAD is suspected in patients with DFI wounds, doppler ultrasonography should be performed by an experienced physician. Direct angiography is performed if PAD is suspected and revascularisation is needed [29]. Revascularisation methods in patients with DFI wounds are endovascular methods and surgical bypass interventions. Revascularisation aims to provide natural pulsatile flow to one of the foot arteries. Preferably, the wound's artery feeding should be selected [30-32].

The standard treatment for ischemic and neuro-ischemic ulcers is femorodistal bypass with autogenous tissue (saphenous vein). If autogenous tissue is unavailable, prosthetic grafts can be used, but they have lower patency rates and are less resistant to infection. In general, surgical bypass is recommended when patients have a life expectancy of more than two years, and a suitable saphenous vein is available. Endovascular treatment is performed if life expectancy is short and there is no suitable autogenous bypass material. Percutaneous transluminal angioplasty may be preferred in high-risk cases with stenosis, or occlusion limited up to 10 cm in length [33].

Infective Endocarditis

The heart consists of 3 layers: epicardium, myocardium, and endocardium from outside to inside. Infection of the endocardial layer is called infective endocarditis. For the development of infective endocarditis, independently affected by different host factors:

1. Predisposing cardiac condition
2. Nonbacterial thrombotic endocarditis (NBTE)
3. Transient bacteremia: Bacterial infestation in NBTE
4. The maturation of vegetation

Intact valve endothelium is resistant to bacterial attachment. Turbulent flow in congenital cardiac abnormalities can cause trauma to the endothelium. Scarring or calcification of the valve in rheumatic valvular diseases or the elderly may result in endothelial damage. Degenerative valvular diseases occur in approximately half of the patients over 60 years of age, which may explain the increasing frequency of infective endocarditis (IE) in the elderly [34, 35].

In the pathogenesis of IE, mechanical damage to the endocardium or inflammation plays a role.

In the mechanically damaged endocardium, NBTE occurs first. Then, with transient bacteremia, bacteria settle in the lesion. Finally, vegetation is formed by the overgrowth of bacteria together with fibrinogen and platelets.

Transient bacteremia occurs in tooth brushing and chewing cases, but the intact endothelium is resistant to bacterial colonisation and thrombus formation. Microbial adherence is a critical step in the pathogenesis of endocarditis and involves complex interactions between microbial surface proteins and host extracellular matrix molecules. Virulent bacteria such as S. aureus may also attach to the intact endothelium and cause acute endocarditis. In response to inflammation in endothelial cells, integrins emerge and bind to fibronectin and form aggregates. Bacteria bind to fibronectin via their binding proteins and are recruited into the endothelial cell. After internalization by endothelial cells, a proinflammatory chemokine response is stimulated. This causes the release of tissue factors and cytokines from endothelial cells. Infected endothelial cells with bacterial products may be lysed, or the bacterium may persist within the cell by changing to a small colony variant phenotype. S. aureus can cause IE in heart valves that are not "normally" damaged and can enter the cell and progress into the tissue depths by causing aggressive tissue damage thanks to its exoproteins. In this way, intracellular S. aureus, which can be pathogenic, is from the host defence system and protected from antibiotics' effects [36].

Endocarditis remains a therapeutic challenge despite effective antibiotic therapy. Two events are significant in the pathogenesis of endocarditis: Endothelial damage and the inability of the endothelium to maintain local antithrombotic function. As a result, vegetation and local thrombosis occur. The tissue factor is thought to play an essential role in this process [37]. The underlying mechanisms by which endothelial damage is induced and vegetation formation occurs have yet to be fully elucidated. However, many details of the pathogenesis of endocarditis need to be further investigated in the future.

Association between Chronic Odontogenic Infection and Cardiovascular Disease Risk

Several studies have described an association between chronic odontogenic infection and cardiovascular disease. Of importance is that intensive periodontal treatment appears to result in improvement of endothelial function, as well as in oral health. The mechanisms by which chronic periodontitis predisposes to coronary heart disease are not well understood, but an adverse effect of systemic inflammation on endothelial function may play a role. In addition to local infection, other factors may contribute to systemic inflammation, including intermittent bacteremia and the release of bacterial endotoxins of oral origin into the bloodstream. This effect can be induced by chewing [38].

Meningococcemia

Meningococcemia is a bacteremia and sepsis syndrome caused by *Neisseria meningitidis* with fever, petechiae, purpura, and hemodynamic instability.

Endothelial injury is central to many clinical features of meningococcemia, including increased vascular permeability, pathologic changes in vascular tonus, loss of thrombo-resistance, intravascular coagulation, and myocardial dysfunction. Leakage of fluid and electrolytes into the tissues from capillaries (capillary leak syndrome) leads to hypovolemia, tissue edema, and pulmonary oedema. Initial compensation results in vasoconstriction and tachycardia, although cardiac output eventually decreases. At the same time, resuscitation fluids may restore circulating volume but can continue to increase tissue edema. Shock in meningococcal septicemia appears to be attributable to a combination of factors, including hypovolemia, which results from the capillary leak syndrome secondary to endothelial injury, and myocardial depression, which is driven by hypovolemia, hypoxia, metabolic derangements. The skin lesions cause widespread endothelial necrosis and occlusion of small vessels in the dermis and subcutaneous tissues with a neutrophilic infiltrate. These mechanisms can be common and deadly in infections with diffuse endothelial involvement (e.g., meningococcemia). Inflammation can cause dysfunction of the vascular endothelium, accompanied by cell death and loss of barrier integrity, giving rise to subcutaneous and body-cavity oedema [39, 40].

Conclusion

Tissue vascularisation can be impaired in many infectious diseases. For example, microvascular thrombosis can occur in many infectious diseases causing sepsis. It plays an essential role in multiple organ failures and mortality. In COVID-19, endothelial damage occurs through direct and indirect mechanisms. Cytokines, complement activation, activated platelets, and immune cells play a role in indirect damage. The development of targeted therapies will guide the treatment of not only COVID-19 but also many other viral and bacterial infections.

References

[1] Mazurek R., Dave J. M., Chandran R. R., Misra A., Sheikh A. Q., Greif D. M. (2017). Vascular cells in blood vessel wall development and disease. *Advances in Pharmacology*, 78, 323-350.

[2] Libby P., Aikawa M., Jain M. K. (2006). Vascular endothelium and atherosclerosis. *The vascular endothelium* II, 285-306.

[3] Deanfield J. E., Halcox J. P., Rabelink T. J. (2007). Endothelial function and dysfunction: testing and clinical relevance. *Circulation*, 115(10), 1285-1295.

[4] Van der Poll T., Van de Veerdonk F. L., Scicluna B. P., Netea M. G. (2017). The immunopathology of sepsis and potential therapeutic targets. *Nature Reviews Immunology*, 17(7), 407-420.

[5] Boisrame-Helms J., Kremer H., Schini-Kerth V., Meziani F. Endothelial Dysfunction in Sepsis. *Curr. Vasc. Pharmacol.* 2013. 18;11(2):150–60.

[6] Frey E. A., Brett Finlay B. Lipopolysaccharide induces apoptosis in a bovine endothelial cell line via a soluble CD14 dependent pathway. *Microb. Pathog*. 1998. 1;24(2):101–9.

[7] Robaye B., Mosselmans R., Fiers W., Dumont J. E., Galand P. Tumor necrosis factor induces apoptosis (programmed cell death) in normal endothelial cells in vitro. *Am. J. Pathol.* 1991. 138(2):447.

[8] Kirkebøen K. A., Strand O. A. The role of nitric oxide in sepsis – an overview. *Acta Anaesthesiol. Scand.* 1999;43(3):275–88. doi/full/10.1034/j.1399-6576.1999.430307.x

[9] Duffy M. J., Mullan B. A., Craig T. R., Shyamsundar, M., MacSweeney R. E., Thompson, G., McAuley, D. F. (2011). Impaired endothelium-dependent vasodilatation is a novel predictor of mortality in intensive care. *Critical care medicine*, 39(4), 629-635.

[10] Joffre J., Hellman J., Ince C., Ait-Oufella H. Endothelial responses in sepsis. *Am. J. Respir. Crit. Care Med*. 2020;202(3):361–70.

[11] Darwish I., Conrad Liles W. Emerging therapeutic strategies to prevent infection-related microvascular endothelial activation and dysfunction. *Virulence*. 2013;4(6).

[12] Zhu J., Ji P., Pang J., Zhong Z., Li H., He C., Zhao C. (2020). Clinical characteristics of 3062 COVID-19 patients: a meta-analysis. *Journal of medical virology*, 92(10), 1902-1914.

[13] Huang R., Zhu L., Xue L., Liu L., Yan X., Wang J., Wu C. (2020). Clinical findings of patients with coronavirus disease 2019 in Jiangsu province, China: A retrospective, multi-center study. *PLoS neglected tropical diseases*, 14(5), e0008280.

[14] Gupta A., Madhavan M. V., Sehgal K., Nair N., Mahajan S., Sehrawat T. S., Landry D. W. (2020). Extrapulmonary manifestations of COVID-19. *Nature medicine,* 26(7), 1017-1032.

[15] Helms J., Severac F., Merdji H., Clere-Jehl R., François B., Mercier E., Meziani F. (2020). Performances of disseminated intravascular coagulation scoring systems in septic shock patients. *Annals of intensive care*, 10(1), 1-7.

[16] Chocron R., Duceau B., Gendron N., Ezzouhairi N., Khider L., Trimaille A., Smadja D. M. (2021). D-dimer at hospital admission for COVID-19 are associated with in-hospital mortality, independent of venous thromboembolism: Insights from a French multicenter cohort study. *Archives of Cardiovascular Diseases*, 114(5), 381-393.

[17] Godo S, Shimokawa H. Endothelial Functions. *Arterioscler. Thromb. Vasc. Biol.* 2017; 37(9):e108–14.

[18] Thachil J., Juffermans N. P., Ranucci M., Connors J. M., Warkentin T. E., Ortel T. L., Levy J. H. (2020). ISTH DIC subcommittee communication on anticoagulation in COVID-19. *Journal of Thrombosis and Haemostasis*, 18(9), 2138-2144.

[19] Jonmarker S., Hollenberg J., Dahlberg M., Stackelberg O., Litorell J., Everhov Å. H., Cronhjort M. (2020). Dosing of thromboprophylaxis and mortality in critically ill COVID-19 patients. *Critical Care*, 24(1), 1-10.

[20] Asakura H., Ogawa H. COVID-19-associated coagulopathy and disseminated intravascular coagulation. *Int. J. Hematol*. 2021;113(1):45–57.

[21] Guo Y., Korteweg C., McNutt M. A., Gu J. Pathogenetic mechanisms of severe acute respiratory syndrome. *Virus Res*. 2008;133(1):4–12.

[22] Hamming I., Timens W., Bulthuis M. L. C., Lely A. T., Navis G. J., Van Goor H. Tissue distribution of ACE2 protein, the functional receptor for SARS coronavirus. A first step in understanding SARS pathogenesis. *J. Pathol*. 2004;203(2):631–7.

[23] Ding Y., Wang H., Shen H., Li Z., Geng J., Han H., Yao K. (2003). The clinical pathology of severe acute respiratory syndrome (SARS): a report from China. *The Journal of Pathology: A Journal of the Pathological Society of Great Britain and Ireland*, 200(3), 282-289.

[24] Alexiadou K., Doupis J. Management of Diabetic Foot Ulcers. *Diabetes Therapy*. 2012;3(1):1–15.

[25] Brem H., Tomic-Canic M. Cellular and molecular basis of wound healing in diabetes. *J. Clin. Invest*. 2007;117(5):1219–1222.

[26] Jörgens K., Stoll S. J., Pohl J., Fleming T. H., Sticht C., Nawroth P. P., Kroll J. (2015). High tissue glucose alters intersomitic blood vessels in zebrafish via methylglyoxal targeting the VEGF receptor signaling cascade. *Diabetes*, 64(1), 213-225.

[27] Liu Z., Hu L., Zhang T., Xu H., Li H., Yang Z., Deng Z. (2020). PKCβ increases ROS levels leading to vascular endothelial injury in diabetic foot ulcers. *American Journal of Translational Research*, 12(10), 6409.

[28] Laing T., Hanson R., Chan F., Bouchier-Hayes D. The role of endothelial dysfunction in the pathogenesis of impaired diabetic wound healing: A novel therapeutic target? *Med. Hypotheses*. 2007;69(5):1029–31.

[29] Moneta G. L., Yeager R. A., Lee R. W., Porter J. M. Noninvasive localization of arterial occlusive disease: A comparison of segmental Doppler pressures and arterial duplex mapping. *J. Vasc. Surg*. 1993;17(3):578–82.

[30] Hinchliffe R. J., Andros G., Apelqvist J., Bakker K., Fiedrichs S., Lammer J., Schaper N. C. (2012). A systematic review of the effectiveness of revascularization of the ulcerated foot in patients with diabetes and peripheral arterial disease. *Diabetes/metabolism research and reviews*, 28, 179-217.

[31] Söderström M., Albäck A., Biancari F., Lappalainen K., Lepäntalo M., Venermo M. Angiosome-targeted infrapopliteal endovascular revascularization for treatment of diabetic foot ulcers. *J. Vasc. Surg*. 2013;57(2):427–35.

[32] Azuma N., Uchida H., Kokubo T., Koya A., Akasaka N., Sasajima T. Factors influencing wound healing of critical ischaemic foot after bypass surgery: is the angiosome important in selecting bypass target artery? *Eur. J. Vasc. Endovasc. Surg*. 2012;43(3):322–8.

[33] Conte M. S. (2010). Challenges of distal bypass surgery in patients with diabetes: patient selection, techniques, and outcomes. *Journal of the American Podiatric Medical Association*, 100(5), 429-438.

[34] Croft L. B., Donnino R., Shapiro R., Indes J., Fayngersh A., Squire A., Goldman M. E. (2004). Age-related prevalence of cardiac valvular abnormalities warranting infectious endocarditis prophylaxis. *The American journal of cardiology*, 94(3), 386-389.

[35] Widmer E., Que Y. A., Entenza J. M., Moreillon P. New concepts in the pathophysiology of infective endocarditis. *Curr. Infect. Dis. Rep.* 2006;8(4):271–9.

[36] Salgado-Pabón W., Breshears L., Spaulding A. R., Merriman J. A., Stach C. S., Horswill A. R., Schlievert P. M. (2013). Superantigens are critical for *Staphylococcus aureus* Infective endocarditis, sepsis, and acute kidney injury. *MBio*, 4(4), e00494-13.

[37] Loughman A., Fitzgerald J. R., Brennan M. P., Higgins J., Downer R., Cox D., Foster T. J. (2005). Roles for fibrinogen, immunoglobulin and complement in platelet activation promoted by *Staphylococcus aureus* clumping factor A. *Molecular microbiology*, 57(3), 804-818.

[38] Koletsi D., Iliadi A., Tzanetakis G. N., Vavuranakis M., Eliades T. Cardiovascular Disease and Chronic Endodontic Infection. Is There an Association? A Systematic Review and Meta-Analysis. *Int. J. Environ. Res. Public Health.* 2021;18(17).

[39] Coureuil M., Join-Lambert O., Lécuyer H., Bourdoulous S., Marullo S., Nassif X. Pathogenesis of Meningococcemia. *Cold Spring Harb. Perspect. Med.* 2013;3(6).

[40] Nieuwland R., Berckmans R. J., McGregor S., Böing A. N., Th. M. Romijn F. P., Westendorp R. G., Sturk A. (2000). Cellular origin and procoagulant properties of microparticles in meningococcal sepsis. *Blood, The Journal of the American Society of Hematology*, 95(3), 930-935.

Chapter 5

Vascularization in COVID-19 Sepsis

Zubeyir Sivrikaya*, MD

Trabzon Kanuni Training and Research Hospital, Department of Anesthesiology, Trabzon, Turkey

Abstract

Sepsis; It causes health professionals to experience economic and medical problems in managing the disease, as both mortality and morbidity rates are high and hospital infections are common. Entry of the SARS-CoV-2 virus into the human body is most commonly via droplet to the upper respiratory tract. It enters the host cell by using angiotensin-converting enzyme 2 (ACE-2) receptors, which are found at high rates in the lung's alveoli, myocyte cells of the heart, vascular endothelial cells, and many cells. This virus has a high affinity for the host cell; it is known to act by using the ACE-2 receptor and binding with its spike protein. The SARS-CoV-2 virus has a high affinity for ACE-2, especially in alveolar epithelial type II and endothelial cells. The virus has been shown to attack and damage these cells directly. SARS-CoV-2 uses virus spike protein and binds to the ACE-2 receptor, injuring alveolar vascular epithelial cells, macrophages, and monocytes.

Many studies have examined and tried to define the mechanisms of coagulopathy developing due to COVID-19 sepsis. However, the existing mechanisms have been insufficient to explain the coagulopathy that occurs. Unfortunately, the treatment strategies related to these did not give satisfactory results. Although we did not leave it behind ultimately, we left the moderate and severe COVID-19 disease behind at the time I wrote the chapter. However, we may encounter different pandemics in the future. We must be prepared to eliminate such epidemics with the least damage.

---

* Corresponding Author's Email: drzbyrs@hotmail.com.

In: Vascularization and Its Role in Medicine and Tissue Engineering
Editors: Emre Bulbul and Murat Oguz Ozilhan
ISBN: 979-8-89113-041-8

Keywords: sepsis, COVID-19, endothelial dysfunction, microvascular thrombosis, vascular endothelial cells

Introduction

Sepsis was first described in the early 1990s, and the definition has been updated again by the Surviving Sepsis Campaign [1]. In addition, in the Third International Consensus Sepsis report published in 2016 by the Society of Critical-Care Medicine (SCCM) and the European Society of Intensive Care Medicine (ESICM), It has been defined as "life-threatening organ dysfunction resulting from a host response" [2].

Sepsis causes health professionals to experience economic and medical problems managing the disease, as high mortality and morbidity rates and hospital infections are typical. It is a complicated process for patients and their relatives. It is a global health problem [3]. The syndrome that forces countries seriously in economic terms. Sepsis and septic shock are among the most common causes of death, especially in surgical and internal medicine intensive care units [4, 5].

Definition

Sepsis is a life-threatening, difficult-to-treat disease that causes the human organism to react with complex mechanisms against the current infection. Septic shock is defined as a mean arterial pressure below 65 mmHg despite adequate fluid resuscitation and lactate levels >2 mmol/L and the need for vasopressor therapy in patients with sepsis. It is reported that septic shock is associated with more than 40% mortality [6].

The Third International Consensus Definitions considers that severe and critically ill patients meet the diagnostic criteria for sepsis and septic shock and recommends using the term 'viral sepsis' for these patients [7, 8].

Expanded Infection Prevalence in Intensive Care II, which investigated the etiology of sepsis, determined that the most common infections were 64% in the lungs, 20% in the abdomen, and 15% in the bloodstream. Gram-negative bacteria are the most common pathogens (62%), followed by gram-positive cocci (47%) and fungi (19%) [9].

Thrombosis; is a state of clot adhesion that occurs with cells such as platelets, leukocytes, and erythrocytes in the vascular endothelial circulation and is tried to be explained by various mechanisms; The resulting clot mass is called a thrombus. Thrombosis can have both physiological and pathological consequences [10].

Coagulation and inflammation are closely related events. They work in conjunction with each other due to injury and various pathogenicities [11, 12]. Inflammation; We can think of it as a natural first response of immunity to tissue damage caused by infection or trauma. As a result, the recognition of the pathogen by the immune system, the assembly of immune cells, the immune response to the threat, and homeostasis occur [13].

Vascular endothelial cell activation and its pathological functioning are critical in developing sepsis [14-17]. In non-pathological conditions, damage to vascular endothelial cells results in an inflammatory effect, and substances such as von Willebrand Factor (vWF), which are responsible for the adhesion of damaged cells, are released into the circulation. In addition, microvascular endothelial cells are further damaged due to virus-mediated inflammatory metabolites and cytokines (such as IL-1α and IFN) damage to epithelial cells [18].

Platelets are important immune cells in the vascular endothelial system. It is known that they have essential roles in vascular endothelial cell damage and proinflammatory conditions as a result of their activation [19]. Many factors, such as platelet surface receptors, immune regulatory chemokines, cytokines, and secretion of growth factors (GFs), are involved in the fulfillment of the functions and properties of platelets [20].

Platelets are of great importance in the pathogenesis of COVID-19 disease. However, there are still many unknown and unexplained points in their role in inflammation and coagulopathy [18]. With inflammation, platelets, monocytes, endothelial cells, and tissue factor (TF) are stimulated, resulting in fibrinolysis. Together, anticoagulant molecules fail to do their job (for example, through changes in thrombomodulin, Protein C and S, and tissue factor pathway inhibitor levels), and they cause thrombosis [21, 22]. Activated protein C, a potent anticoagulant, exhibits profibrinolytic and anti-inflammatory properties, is significantly impaired in vascular sepsis, and is effective in coagulation [23].

A “cytokine storm” may sometimes occur due to the immune system's overreaction to inflammation [24]. Hyperinflammation and hypercoagulation are likely due to cytokine storms [25]. Cytokines and chemokines are induced, triggered by the binding of the COVID-19 virus to angiotensin-converting enzyme 2 (ACE-2) receptors on alveolar epithelial cells. Chemokines; It causes monocytes, macrophages, neutrophils, natural killer cells, dendritic cells, and adaptive immune cells (CD4+, CD8+ T cells) to infiltrate the infected area [26]. They may also contribute to cytokine storms due to overstimulation in severe COVID-19 patients [27, 28].

In simple COVID-19 infection, fever, hypotension, decreased urine output, and thrombocytopenia is the most common clinical findings in sepsis. It can seriously affect the vascular system, especially the microvascular system. If the necessary precautions are not taken or treated, respiratory failure, renal failure, and coagulation disorders occur. Hypotension unresponsive to treatment develops [29]. In a study, in cases of pneumonia due to COVID-19 disease, it has been suggested that there is a pauci-inflammatory septal capillary injury caused by a critical membrane attack complex and accumulation of complement lectin pathway activators in microvascular cells [30].

Epidemiology

Although many microorganisms, such as bacteria, viruses, and fungi, can cause sepsis, bacteria are the most common. Multiple microorganisms are responsible for more than half of sepsis cases [31]. Infections that cause sepsis are generally respiratory system, gastrointestinal system, urinary system-related infections, and bacteremia. The effects of toxins of bacteria or viruses can be detected in nearly half of the detected micro-organisms, and it is known that gram-negative bacteria are responsible for 60%. It is thought that gram-positive bacteria are responsible for the other 40% [4, 5]. It is known that inflammation occurring during sepsis can trigger thrombosis. This coagulopathy, which is caused by the effect of the human immune system, is called immunothrombosis [32].

Incidence

According to the report of The Global Burden of Disease Study in 2017, 48.9 million sepsis cases that can be detected worldwide have been reported. It is estimated that there are 11 million deaths due to sepsis [33]. In another study conducted in 2020, the incidence of death due to sepsis and septic shock was reported as 35.3% and 52% [34]. A further study shows that more than 20% of patients who survive after sepsis dies within the next two years [35].

Advanced age, immunosuppression, and multidrug-resistant infection are among the incidences of Sepsis [36, 37]. It also shows differences between races. When we look at the age groups of sepsis patients, we see that 60-85% consists of patients over the age of 65; with the increase in aging in parallel with the increase in population, we can expect that the rate of sepsis may increase in the following years [4, 38-40].

In the early recognition and early treatment of sepsis, the mortality rates are reported to be highly variable, such as 20-80% [41]. Evaluation of Sepsis-Related Organ Failure (SOFA) scoring is still an indicator of sepsis-related mortality. The central nervous system Glasgow coma score, respiratory PaO 2 /FiO 2, the amount of vasoactive drug required to prevent cardiovascular system hypotension, liver bilirubin level, renal serum creatinine or urine output, and coagulation platelet concentration parameters are used, and a score of 1 to 4 is given. The SCCM and the ESICM approve the SOFA score as a tool to identify patients at risk of dying from sepsis [8, 42]. A score of 9 in scoring was associated with more than 33% mortality in multicenter studies [43, 44].

SOFA is used in the early detection of organ failure and is generally preferred for patients hospitalized in the intensive care unit. SOFA score remains a valuable parameter in sepsis due to COVID-19 infection [45]. The quick SOFA scoring is the most common and easy-to-use scoring tool that helps assess the risk of death from sepsis [8, 46]. Respiration rate, systolic blood pressure, and level *of consciousness or new confusion are used for quick SOFA scoring.*

The score obtained indicates the mortality risk of sepsis and the urgency of the response:

- 0 to 4 – low risk (3 points on any parameter low-moderate)
- 5 to 6 – medium risk
- seven or more - high risk [47]

Septic shock is a clinical subform of sepsis with high mortality, progressing with severe hypotension [8]. Sepsis and septic shock can start as a severe acute respiratory system disease that progresses to multiple organ failure and death at serious rates. It is a disease that affects many organ systems, filling intensive care units, suppressing immunity, damaging the vascular endothelial system, and affecting the coagulation systems significantly [48, 49].

In a study conducted in 94 centers and 132 *intensive care units* (ICU) in Turkey, 1499 patients were evaluated, the septic shock rate was approximately 7%, and the mortality rate was approximately 75.9%. This important study in our country shows us the seriousness and importance of sepsis [50].

Another clinical outcome that can be seen in sepsis may be a multi-organ dysfunction syndrome (MODS). Generally, the increase in incidence is correlated with the increase in mortality. The most significant risk for MODS is respiratory failure with prolonged mechanical ventilator requirements [51-53].

When we look at sepsis risk factors, nosocomial infections occur at a rate of approximately 50 percent in intensive care hospitalizations and have a very high risk for sepsis [54]. The risk of sepsis is high for patients over the age of 65, and independently of sepsis, it is a significant risk factor for advanced age mortality [55]. Any disease or medication that causes immunosuppression poses a severe risk for sepsis. Obesity and diabetes, especially infections related to them, are among the significant problems of recent years and pose a multifaceted risk for sepsis [56]. Cancer, genetic factors, nutritional disorders, and socio-economic risks are among the important risk factors for sepsis [57-60].

COVID-19 infection caused secondary infections, sepsis, and death by affecting the endothelial structure, which is the vascular structure of the respiratory system, through various mechanisms. Therefore, sepsis and mortality due to COVID-19 have become a considerable risk **[61].**

COVID-19 Sepsis and Vascular Mechanism

It is the disease caused by the SARS-CoV-2 virus, which constitutes the main agenda of the whole world in COVID-19. Severe COVID-19 patients meet the diagnostic criteria for sepsis and have similarities and differences with sepsis caused by pathogens other than the SARS-CoV-2 virus. Patients with severe COVID-19 most suffer severely from multi-organ failure characterized by sepsis [62].

Vascular endothelial cells, the immune system, inflammation, and vascular tone play a critical role in regulating and maintaining vascular homeostasis by many mechanisms in healthy humans [63, 64]. In endothelial cells in a healthy human organism, the coagulation system functions smoothly without causing thrombosis. Thus, the blood flow is kept under physiological control [65].

Vascular endothelial cells are the most critical structure covering the inner surface of the entire vascular and lymphatic systems. An adult human organism weighs more than 100 g and has a surface area of more than 3000 square meters. In total, there are more than one trillion endothelial cells in an adult human [66, 67].

The vascular endothelial glycocalyx structure is significant in endothelial function. The pathological loss of the glycocalyx structure impairs the endothelial function, which results in tissue or organ dysfunction. The endothelial surface layer is densely coexisting with the most common glucosamine glycans and substances called heparan sulfate (HS). Many pathogens, including the SARS-CoV-2 virus, use glycans for initial interaction with cells [68, 69]. We can see the presence of HS in the bloodstream as a disruption of the endothelial barrier layer [70].

In addition, the main critical tasks of vascular endothelial cells;

- In the control of the passage through the vascular system, especially the nutrients required for tissues and cells,
- In balancing the pro-inflammatory and anti-inflammatory mediators, pro-coagulant and anti-coagulant activities,
- In the renewal and maturation of vascular structures (in neovascularization),
- In the healthy development of organs,
- In the flawless functioning of acquired and acquired immunity,
- They are also critical in realizing programmed death with circulating vascular cells [71, 72].

It may begin as symptoms such as fever, weakness, headache, confusion, cough, myalgia, and hypotension. We should not forget that the disease may progress to severe disease states such as systemic inflammatory response syndrome, acute respiratory distress syndrome (ARDS), disseminated intravascular coagulation (DIC), multiple organ failure, sepsis, and septic shock [73].

Many serious infections; In conditions such as hyperinflammation, hemostatic balance is not expected to work in harmony., coagulation disorder, and thrombosis. With inflammation, Activation of coagulation, impaired fibrin destruction by increased intravascular fibrin formation and deposition, and ultimately DIC [74, 75].

Entry of the SARS-CoV-2 virus into the human body is most commonly via droplet to the upper respiratory tract [76]. It enters the host cell by using ACE-2 receptors, which are found at high rates in the lung's alveoli, myocyte cells of the heart, vascular endothelial cells, and many cells [77]. This virus has a high affinity for the host cell; it is known to act by using the ACE-2 receptor and binding with its spike protein [78].

The SARS-CoV-2 virus has a high affinity for ACE-2, especially in alveolar epithelial type II and endothelial cells. The virus has been shown to attack and damage these cells [79] directly. SARS-CoV-2 uses virus spike protein and binds to the ACE-2 receptor, injuring alveolar vascular epithelial cells, macrophages, and monocytes. Protein receptor binding; causes platelet aggregation and triggers immunity [80].

The etiology of coagulopathy seen in COVID-19 disease has yet to be clarified. It is known that it is caused by various pathologies between the immune system, vascular endothelium, coagulation system, and SARS-CoV-2 virus [81]. Endothelial damage caused by vascular endothelial cell activation results in microvascular damage and thrombosis. This results from abnormal coagulopathy observed in COVID-19 patients and are thought to be an essential process that progresses to morbidity and mortality, such as multi-organ MODS [79].

It has been proven that the SARS-CoV-2 virus directly envelops vascular endothelial cells, causing cellular damage and endothelial dysfunction. Many clinicians think that vascular endothelial damage, microvascular inflammation, and endothelial exocytosis/endotheliitis play a critical role in the pathogenesis of ARDS and organ failure in severe COVID-19 patients [82, 83].

Hyper-proliferation and reduction in vasodilation, proinflammatory events, and pro-coagulation severely contribute to the formation of endothelial dysfunction [84, 85]. Coagulation disorders progressing to a mortal state, such as ARDS and severe sepsis, are a condition that we frequently observe in the course of COVID-19 disease.

Obstructive thromboinflammatory syndrome (MicroCLOTS); is a disease characterized by a thrombotic state seen in the microvascular structures of the lung. Diffuse thromboinflammatory events are seen in endothelial cells during this disease [86]. MicroCLOTS has been defined as an atypical form of ARDS, which can also be observed in the microvascular structures of the lung in the course of severe COVID-19 disease [86].

Thromboembolic severe events have been experienced due to coagulopathy in many patients, particularly those due to infection from severe covid-19 disease. Intravascular coagulation of DIC-like conditions or DIC may also develop due to pathologies in this coagulation system [87].

The International Society on Thrombosis and Haemostasis states that sepsis-induced coagulopathy causes less coagulopathy than DIC, but worsening may occur [88-90].

The clinic of venous thromboembolism usually progresses silently, and in many patients, the first sign is sudden fatal pulmonary thromboembolism [91]. These complications often occur in hospitalized COVID-19 patients and can lead to potentially fatal diseases such as pulmonary thromboembolism and deep vein thrombosis [92].

The high prevalence of deep vein thrombosis has been reported to us as associated with adverse outcomes of COVID-19 disease [93]. The early emergence of coagulation problems in COVID-19 may cause asymptomatic deep-vein thrombosis and may be associated with a poor prognosis [94].

According to the results of a recent meta-analysis, it was determined that the rate of venous thromboembolism (VTE) was 25%, and this incidence increased in patients who needed mechanical ventilation [95]. Other studies have shown a 35-45% higher risk of VTE in critically ill COVID-19 patients [96, 97].

In platelet activation with the release of cytokines and growth factors (GF). These processes are known to increase the risk of VTE [18]. In addition, arterial thromboembolism, which can be seen in patients with COVID-19, is a severe disease that can prevent the functions of essential organs [98]. In one study, high numbers of VTE and arterial thromboembolism were noted from the beginning of the disease [99]. Arterial thromboembolism occurring in hyperinflammatory states related to SARS-CoV 2 virus is a risk factor that can be serious [100].

Another event contributing to thrombosis formation is the SARS-COV 2 viral endotoxin-induced expression of TF and plasminogen activator inhibitor-1 (PAI-1) in vascular endothelial cells; TF and PAI-1 activate protease-activated receptors (PAR). Thrombosis formation is stimulated due to PAR increase [101].

Severe SARS-CoV-2 virus infection produces endothelial cell dysfunction with detrimental effects on vascular endothelial cells (VEC), resulting in a disease characterized by hyperinflammation [102]. Almost all cells have TF in their membranes. TF is released from endothelial cells damaged by various experiments. For example, it can be released by monocytes and endothelial cells due to inflammation. TF is found in a compound with factor 7, generally found in the bloodstream. Activation of this compound and reaching the surface of platelets is a critical requirement for the initiation of coagulation [103].

Polyphosphate molecules produced by pathogens can also induce thromboinflammation via monocytes, macrophages, and TF by stimulating inflammation [88, 104].

The resulting inflammatory state is caused by VEC-derived protein C, thrombomodulin, and TF pathway inhibitors. Moreover, an increase in thrombus formation is observed with the deterioration of the anticoagulant response mechanism. The effect of plasminogen activator inhibitor-1 (PAI-1) released from VEC also inhibits fibrinolysis [65]. These events also contribute to thrombus formation.

The main factors causing VEC dysfunction are; decreased nitric oxide production, increased reactive oxygen species production decreased anticoagulant effect, and increased dipeptidyl peptidase-4 and vWF, TF, intercellular adhesion molecule-1, E-selectin and P-selectin.

It has been reported that early production of IL-1α, a proinflammatory cytokine that can be released from endothelial cells, activated platelets, and monocyte cells, provides a bridge between coagulation and inflammation [105, 106]. Another important effect of IL-1α is the infiltration of granulocytes and its contribution to the formation of thrombosis due to inflammation [107].

The affected VEC layer becomes procoagulant and antifibrinolytic. It is associated with the release of vWF by VEC activation and the release of thrombomodulin into the blood. High levels of mediators in the blood are closely related to the morbidity and mortality of the disease. For these reasons, vWF and thrombomodulin play a crucial role in coagulation [108]. The normal function of vWF is the attachment of platelets to the damaged area, accelerating thrombus formation on collagen surfaces [109, 110].

During the course of this disease, as a result of the overreaction of the immune system, what we call the hyper-inflammatory response is observed. In excessive amounts, the hyper-inflammatory effect results in the release of mediators such as TNF-α, IL-1β, IL-8, and IL-6. In addition, hyper-cytokinemia may occur, in which inflammation can be exacerbated by other pro-inflammatory mediators. As a result of all these events, severe hypotension, leakage from the vascular space (tissue edema), MODS, ARDS, and death may occur [13, 111]. It is known to mediate the increase of IL-6 and the coagulation of TNF-α and IL-1 cytokines in patients with sepsis caused by COVID-19 [112].

The pathophysiology of hypercytokinemia, which may occur as a result of COVID-19 disease, may appear as a decrease in lymphocytes due to apoptosis in the spleen and lungs. However, it has similarities with the disease caused by the influenza virus, characterized by large amounts of macrophages, neutrophils, and proinflammatory cytokines [113].

Numerous in vitro studies in recent years have shown that VEC apoptosis occurs in response to bacterial toxins and proinflammatory cytokines. *VEC apoptosis has been demonstrated in several in-vivo studies* [114-116]. VEC apoptosis has been demonstrated in several in-vivo studies [117-119]. Studies in patients who died from sepsis-induced ARDS provided evidence of VEC apoptosis [120].

Pathologies occurring in VEC can be attributed to ischemia-induced stroke caused by SARS -CoV 2 infection [121] and even shown that it can cause a fetal intracerebral hemorrhage [122]. Some autopsy series have also shown edema and neuronal degeneration in the brain [123]. Cerebral petechial hemorrhages and microthrombus formation were also observed in some series. In such studies, endothelium and apoptosis in the vascular structures of the brain, together with lymphocyte and monocyte infiltration in VEC, have been detected [124].

In the case of COVID-19 disease-associated coagulopathy, hypo-fibrinolysis and heparin resistance may occur [125-128]. Death of capillary VECs, damage to the intercellular junction, hydrolysis, and shedding of the glycocalyx and VEC cadherin molecule causes an increase in vessel permeability [129]. Thus tissue edema occurs.

In cases of ARDS, severe sepsis, multi-organ failure, and mortality caused by COVID-19, we see those immune system mediators such as interleukin (IL)-1β, IL-6, and tumor necrosis factor-α (TNF-α) increase through VEC [130]. IL-6 levels continue to rise as the disease progresses in severe cases [131].

In severe COVID-19 disease, elevations in IL-6 and D- dimer levels are detected. Tocilizumab (anti-IL-6) is used for the cytokine storm seen during the disease. Therefore, IL-6 levels are essential in treatment and follow-up offers [132]. In a study conducted in 2020, IL-6 and procalcitonin values were shown to be important for the severity of COVID-19 disease [133].

In addition, a recently published multicenter study on 1039 COVID-19 patients determined that the most important parameters as an indicator of the ICU mortality rate were high IL-6, procalcitonin, and CRP values [134]. Elevated IL-6 levels indicate increased platelet activity, fibrinogen-related inflammation, and increased thrombosis [135, 136]. It is also thought that IL-

6 contributes to thrombosis by affecting VEC and monocytes, causing TF expression from these cells [137]. We also see that IL-6 released from VECs increases vascular permeability through vascular endothelial-derived growth factors (VEGF) [138].

C-reactive protein is an acute-phase protein; it is crucial as a biochemical value that can rise in COVID-19 patients [139]. It has gained even more value as a parameter that shows us the probability of an exacerbation in non-serious COVID-19 patients [140]. In a study, CRP and fibrinogen decreased in patients with arterial thromboembolism and deep vein thrombus after treatment [141]. In a study involving 76 patients with COVID-19, it was thought that high CRP and procalcitonin levels might be associated with death [142].

Macrophage inflammatory protein 1α was also detected in COVID-19 patients hospitalized in the ICU [143]. On the other hand, some cytokines such as IL-1β, IL-6, IL-9, IL-17A, modifier growth factor-β (TGF-β), and chemokine ligand 2 were effective in forming thrombosis and stimulating other cytokines [144].

Among the vascular endothelial-derived growth factors, growth factors such as VEGF, insulin growth factor-1, platelet-derived growth factor, and TGF-β have also been found to have essential roles in the pathogenesis of coagulopathy. It has been determined that there are deteriorations in the activities of GFs in severe COVID-19 patients [145]. Studies suggest that the elevation of hepatocyte growth factor, another GF, may indicate the severity and mortality of the disease in COVID-19 patients [146]. In addition, activated VEC releases the P-selectin molecule. vWF causes the secretion of thromboxane A2 procoagulant, inflammatory PAI-1, and antifibrinolytic molecules. This aggravates the formation of thrombosis [147, 148].

We see that fibrinogen levels increase early in the course of COVID-19 disease. For this reason, it is understood that it can be used in the early diagnosis of the disease [149]. Balance changes in the fibrinolytic system and coagulation pathways and damage to the endothelial membrane and pulmonary arteries cause the accumulation of fibrinogen-like coagulation products in the alveoli. For such reasons, TF is stimulated, and fibrin formation occurs [150].

The study of 466 patients showed us that with the severity of the disease, high levels of fibrin degradation products occur [151].

Damaged VECs cause the release of TF, which binds and activates factor VII to initiate the coagulation cascade with thrombin and clot formation at the end of the process [152]. TF is usually found in very low amounts in the circulatory system. With its increase, clotting activation and thrombin formation are induced, resulting in platelet, vascular endothelium, and leukocyte activation. At the same time, cytokine secretion and severe inflammation increase [153, 154].

It is known that there is a significant relationship between the increase in leukocytes and the decrease in lymphocytes (Lymphocytopenia) in many severe COVID-19 patients. In addition, it has been shown that the decrease in lymphocytes is more in young people [155]. Some studies associate the decrease in lymphocyte count with oxygen demand [156].

Lymphocytopenia is a condition that we frequently see in COVID-19 patients. It has been determined that the significant decrease in lymphocyte count increases three times with the aggravation of the disease in severe COVID-19 patients [157]. In addition, lymphopenia has been associated with coagulation disorder and hematological changes in COVID-19 disease [158].

The platelet/lymphocyte ratio (PLR) is significant in severe COVID-19 disease, and it has been documented that an increase in the platelet/lymphocyte ratio is correlated with prolonged disease duration [159]. A study found that thrombocytopenia increased mortality three times in COVID-19 patients with thrombocytopenia [160]. A study of 1476 patients with COVID-19 observed that the risk of death with thrombocytopenia was significantly increased [161].

The neutrophil/lymphocyte ratio is an important prognostic factor in many hematological pathologies, and it has been reported that this ratio is increased in COVID-19 patients [162]. A study conducted on 245 patients with COVID-19 reported that an increase in the neutrophil/lymphocyte ratio could be used to determine the risk [163].

Neutrophils are one of the essential elements of innate immunity. It is one of the factors that cause thrombosis formation by interacting with platelets and VEC. Neutrophils emerging from the vascular bed with increased vascular permeability are the first cells to enter the area of inflammation by diapedesis and chemotaxis. They form the first line of defense against threats entering the body [164, 165].

They also provide intercellular communication, essential in inflammation, by sending signals to other cells [166]. Neutrophils are at the forefront of natural defense, where they induce phagocytosis, degranulation, and formation of neutrophil-derived extracellular traps (NETs) [167]. Neutrophils can trap and kill pathogens using NETs, thus preventing the spread of pathogens into the bloodstream and surrounding tissues [168-170].

As a result of the excessive immune response in COVID-19 patients, platelets can cause coagulation with both increased platelet activity and increased TF activity, as well as increased platelet-monocyte and platelet-neutrophil aggregates that may occur during the NETosis process [171]. Hyperinflammation, microvascular thrombosis, and higher NET levels have been demonstrated in patients with COVID-19 compared to ARDS patients.

The NET formation has been accepted as an indicator of high virulence in COVID -19 patients. NETs can down-regulate their activity to exploit the effects of thrombosis and inflammation proportionally, but this may be impaired in the case of hyperinflammation. NETosis is a form of immune defense that induces trap formation in which regulated neutrophil death traps pathogens and thus prevents further spread. NETs formed by triggering innate immunity can cause cell death, such as apoptosis and necrosis. However, the fact that it occurs at a time and place where it should not be and has a low density causes undesirable results [167].

In the case of sepsis, NET formation may occur with polymorphonuclear leukocyte-platelet interaction. NETs entering the circulation can damage VEC. As a result of these events (NETosis/apoptosis/necrosis), chromatin filaments are exposed. This causes thrombus formation and disturbance in blood flow. This indicates that NETosis increases the occurrence of thrombosis [172].

The neutrophils that most commonly cause NETosis are the neutrophils that are collected at the infection site and have completed their life [173]. NETs also facilitate fibrin polymerization, vWF binding to platelets, platelet adhesion to the damaged site, and erythrocyte retention [174]. Another study proved that venous thrombus formation and dissemination could occur with NET [175, 176]. Due to such reasons, NETs inhibit fibrinolysis and adversely affect coagulation in cases of hyperinflammation [177, 178]. In addition, NETs that come to the area of cellular damage caused by inflammation or other effects can create a prothrombotic environment, inhibit natural anticoagulants, and may cause coagulation factors to come to these areas [179, 180].

Myeloperoxidase (MPO), another neutrophilic enzyme and one of the essential elements of the immune system, has a significant effect on the formation of microthrombus [97]. Also found in vascular endothelial cells ADAMTS-1significantly contribute3 (a disintegrin with a thrombospondin type 1 motif and metalloproteinase 13) and exerts a prothrombotic effect by inhibiting the cleavage of vWF [181]. MPO is thought to exert another prothrombotic activity by forming NETs [182] MPO-DNA levels detected in some COVID-19 patients have been associated with NET formation [183].

This immunothrombotic state is further strengthened by neutrophil cell activation and complement activation triggered by the coagulation system. In addition, factor XIIa, which is involved in the formation of coagulation in the immune system, is effective in thrombosis by stimulating the production of bradykinin and kallikrein [184, 185].

In postmortem studies in severe COVID-19 patients, extensive endothelial cell damage in pulmonary vascular beds, microvascular thrombosis, occlusion in alveolar capillary vascular structures, and neoangiogenesis have been found [186]. One of the mechanisms of microvascular thrombosis that may be specific to COVID-19 is events resulting from the affinity of the virus for ACE-2 receptors expressed in alveolar epithelial type II cells and various extrapulmonary tissues, including endothelial cells. SARS-CoV 2 has been shown to invade the endothelial cell directly. Endothelial cell activation may be a unique mechanism of COVID-19-mediated microvascular injury, thrombosis, and subsequent MODS. These are believed to significantly contribute to coagulopathy, morbidity, and mortality [72]. Some histopathological examinations in COVID-19 patients also revealed extensive alveolar damage due to severe inflammation and thrombotic microangiopathy in the pulmonary vascular structures [187]. In a postmortem series of 11 patients, thrombosis of the pulmonary arteries was demonstrated in all patients [188]. Some postmortem studies observed multiple organ failures due to thrombotic microangiopathy [189, 190]. Microvascular thrombosis has also been reported in the acute phase of multiple organ failures [191].

Macroscopic pulmonary thrombus was demonstrated in approximately 34% of postmortem studies. This thrombus formation during severe COVID-19 infection is known as "immunothrombosis" [192]. A study by Klok et al. on critical COVID-19 patients reported that the combined incidence of DVT, pulmonary embolism (PE), and arterial thrombosis was 31%. In another study, PE was seen in 81% of such patients [193]. In some studies, the occurrence of PE has been described as an essential indicator of mortality for COVID-19 patients even alone [194]. The mortality rate is thought to increase to 30% in untreated PE patients and up to 10-15% in treated patients [195]. In the recently published study, PE was thought to be associated with less severity in patients with COVID-19 than in patients without COVID-19 [196]. In COVID-19 patients who were closely followed and treated, the presence of pulmonary microthrombus was demonstrated in 72% of the autopsy series [197].

The platelet factor 4 (PF4) molecule released by platelet activation in platelets has a crucial role in Ig-G-mediated antibody formation in heparin-induced thrombocytopenia [198, 199]. Binding pathogens and antibodies to PF4 further increase platelet aggregation and thrombosis formation. This mechanism is also noteworthy in sepsis due to COVID-19 [200, 201]. The PF4 molecule has also been blamed for complications defined as vaccine-induced immune thrombotic thrombocytopenia and is also referred to by different names in some studies [202, 203].

An increase in vWF, which is a sign of VEC activation, which we mentioned before, is associated with the severity and mortality of the disease in COVID-19 [108]. Endothelial cell activation is essential for COVID-19-mediated microvascular damage, thrombosis, and subsequent multi-system organ failure. It contributes to coagulopathy formation, morbidity, and mortality [79].

Thrombus seen in the vascular endothelial system was not only seen in diseases caused by SARS-CoV 2 virus but also in diseases caused by SARS-CoV 1 and MERS viruses, which we have seen in previous years [204].

An essential element of severe COVID-19 disease is its resemblance and association with hemophagocytic lymphohistiocytosis disease (HLH). Cytokine storm due to severe disease has significant clinical and laboratory findings similar to HLH. It is thought that conditions such as fever, cytopenia, elevation in liver function tests and ferritin elevations, and ARDS may have developed due to HLH [205, 206].

Laboratory

Coagulation tests are used for follow-up in cases of unexplained bleeding, in patients with a high risk of bleeding, and in patients receiving anticoagulant and antiaggregant therapy. The relevant history and examination findings from patients and their relatives provide important clues regarding the location and follow-up of the hemostatic disorder and guide us for further tests.

Thrombocytopenia

It is the platelet count below $150x10^9$ /µl-mm3 in the complete blood count. Confirming low platelet counts with peripheral smear is essential in terms of misleading results.

Bleeding Time

Bleeding time is prolonged in disorders of the functions of proteins, such as platelet disorders, vWF, and fibrinogen. Von Willebrand disease is the most common inherited disease that prolongs bleeding time.

Platelet Function Tests

When the platelet count is normal, prolonging the bleeding time indicates a problem with platelet functions.

Prothrombin Time (PT)

The essential usage area is to detect deficiencies of FII, FVII, FX, prothrombin, and fibrinogen in the intrinsic and common pathways and to follow up vitamin K antagonist (coumadin) treatment. The increase in PT value helps us with factor deficiencies, factor synthesis deficiencies that can be seen in liver patients. It can help in the proteolytic depletion of factors, coagulation factors, and the presence of antibodies against phospholipids [207].

International Normalized Ratio (INR)

It is a measure used to evaluate the extrinsic and common coagulation pathways. In theory, it helps coagulopathy associated with COVID-19 and assesses liver function [208]. INR prolongation is less significant in the severity of COVID-19 disease and coagulopathy compared to D-dimer elevation [209].

Many studies show a prolongation in PT, INR, and thrombin time parameters in parallel with the severity of COVID-19 [210-215].

Activated Partial Thromboplastin Time (aPTT)

Its prolongation is helpful in cases such as DIC, massive transfusion, liver disease, heparin therapy, or mixing with the sample.

Fibrinogen

It may be low in the presence of substances such as fibrinogen degradation products (inhibiting fibrin polymerization) or in patients receiving fibrinolytic therapy.

Thrombin Time

The most common reason for its increase is the presence of heparin in the blood sample [207].

We see an increase in D-dimer and fibrinogen amounts and minimal increases in PT, aPTT, and platelet counts among the tests we frequently apply when evaluating coagulopathy [88]. It has also been observed that biochemical values such as AST, ALT, and LDH, which also indicate liver damage, are elevated, especially in severe and fatal patients (approximately 49% of all patients admitted to the hospital) [216].

The breakdown of fibrin forms D-dimer. It is also an indicator of coagulation and fibrinolysis [217]. Coagulopathy evaluation in COVID-19 patients includes various coagulation tests and hematological scans such as D-dimer analysis and platelet count. In one study, we see consistently high D-dimer levels associated with disease severity in patients with severe COVID-19 [218].

In COVID-19-associated coagulopathy, significantly elevated D-dimer levels and increased fibrinogen levels are observed, which indicates severe thrombotic status [217]. The coagulation indicators observed in DIC are at normal levels [219]. In another study, elevated D-dimer levels were observed in patients with severe COVID-19, triggered by cytokine storm, resulting in MODS and often death [18].

D-dimers distinguish biochemical parameters from fibrinogen, CRP, ferritin, and other biochemical parameters associated with COVID-19 infection [220-222]. Detected at the time of patient admission to the hospital is associated with mortality in many studies [88, 210, 223]. The increase in D-dimer levels after hospitalization, especially in ICU hospitalizations, can indicate MODS and DIC formation. It is mainly seen with microvascular coagulation rather than bleeding [88].

We frequently encounter situations from laboratory indicators, including lymphopenia, elevated LDH, elevated CRP, increased D-dimer, ferritin, and IL-6 levels. D-dimer and IL-6 levels help us to show the severity of the disease and coagulation disorder. The increase in fibrinogen level in parallel with the increase in IL-6 draws the attention [224]. Considering the increase in D-dimer levels in patients without apparent symptoms, hospitalization and close follow-up are required due to the risk of thrombin formation and thrombosis [211].

Factor VIII and fibrinogen levels in plasma are remarkably elevated in COVID-19 patients. However, natural anticoagulants such as protein C and antithrombin decrease slightly [217]. Thrombocytopenia can be seen in severe COVID-19 patients, although the platelet count does not change in most patients followed [225]. Thrombocytopenia, commonly observed in intravascular thrombosis and DIC, presents an increase in D-dimer elevation and prolonged coagulation times (especially PT) in coagulation activity. Therefore, ischemia and MODS occur due to an obstruction in the vascular system [226].

Treatment

Surviving Sepsis Campaign (SSC) has published a guideline on managing critically ill patients with COVID-19 in ICU. The guideline tells us to use dynamic parameters such as skin temperature, capillary refill time, and serum lactate measurement instead of static parameters to evaluate fluid response. The guideline recommends using balanced crystalloid fluids as fluid support and, if necessary, norepinephrine (noradrenaline) as a first-line vasopressor. In the presence of COVID-19 sepsis and shock, low-dose corticosteroid therapy recommends approximately 200 mg of hydrocortisone per day. Supplemental oxygen is recommended if the peripheral oxygen saturation is less than 92%. More than 75% of inpatients say supplemental oxygen may be needed, and high-flow nasal cannula oxygen therapy may be required if they are not responding to standard oxygen therapy [227]. Early and controlled intubation may be beneficial in minimizing nosocomial infections [228].

Systemic steroid therapy was not routinely recommended at the beginning of the COVID-19 pandemic. As knowledge and experience developed rapidly, the use of steroids became widespread. Finally, anti-inflammatory treatments that suppress immune-induced systemic inflammation and cytokine storm, especially corticosteroids, have become important. A study on the use of corticosteroids in hospitalized patients with ARDS due to COVID-19 reports that the use of corticosteroids may have positive potential benefits in terms of mortality need and duration of mechanical ventilation in patients with ARDS [229].

SCC guidelines recommend using systemic steroids, especially in patients with COVID-19 sepsis and associated ARDS who need mechanical ventilation and are intubated [227].

In the multicenter RECOVERY study, patients who received dexamethasone for an additional ten days of standard care had a lower mortality rate than patients who received standard care. This study was significant only in COVID-19 patients with severe comorbidity and supplemental oxygen requirement. It has been determined that there is no benefit in patients who do not require oxygen support therapy [230].

Some studies have shown us that despite anticoagulant treatment in many COVID-19-related infections, a high rate of thrombus occurs in patients with disease-related pneumonia [231, 232]. In COVID-19 patients who develop ARDS, We should not forget that there may be a cascade of pulmonary inflammation, endothelial damage, and microvascular thrombosis, which may result in death. Although the studies showing that heparin treatment used in such patients reduces the severity of the disease and the risk of death are satisfactory, they are insufficient [233-235].

Heparins or low molecular weight heparins, frequently used in coagulopathy treatment, also have antiviral and anti-inflammatory effects [236]. Although studies show that therapeutic heparin is ineffective in severe COVID-19 patients, randomized controlled studies show that it is beneficial in moderate COVID-19 patients [237, 238]. Recently, the American Society of Hematology and International Society for Thrombosis and Hemostasis guidelines recommend prophylactic anticoagulants in all COVID-19 patients until there is clear evidence that prophylactic anticoagulant use is useless [239].

The prevalence of VTE in patients (81 patients) treated for severe COVID-19 pneumonia at Union Hospital of China was studied. As a result of this study, the increase in D-dimer levels and the prevalence of VTE were reduced by using anticoagulant treatments [240].

In a retrospective study conducted on patients given acetylsalicylic acid (aspirin), which we use as an anti-aggregant, it has been shown that aspirin prophylaxis given one week before or 24 hours after it causes a decrease in mortality [241]. It is vital to prevent cytokine storm and coagulation disorders from resulting in serious cardiovascular complications in severe and mortal COVID-19 patients. For these reasons, it is believed that the severity of the disease and the effects on the cardiovascular system will be avoided by taking advantage of its anti-virus replication, anti-platelet aggregation, anticoagulant, and anti-inflammatory effects by using aspirin. In addition, it is expected to reduce and prevent the incidence of severe cases and the length of hospital stay by using it in the early period [242].

Statins have satisfactory results in the treatment of COVID-19-associated vascular endothelial pathologies. It is thought that it may cause improvements in endothelial cell functions by acting on vascular endothelial nitric oxide synthase (eNOS) [243]. Evidence shows that statins have immunomodulatory and anti-inflammatory activities [244]. In a retrospective study, a decrease in mortality was observed in COVID-19 patients using statins [245].

Tocilizumab, an IL-6 receptor antagonist, was thought to be an excellent candidate therapy for survival in severe COVID-19 patients [246, 247]. Scientists conducting a study called REMAP-CAP also reported that they achieved similar results between the IL-6 antagonist's tocilizumab and sarilumab in critically ill COVID-19 patients who need organ supportive care [238].

A potentially effective anti-inflammatory drug for severe COVID-19 patients is anakinra, an IL-1 inhibitor. IL-1 is a proinflammatory cytokine and is known to be associated with severe COVID-19. Several studies have shown us a reduction in mortality and the need for mechanical ventilators after anakinra therapy. No serious adverse events were reported [248, 249].

Baricitinib, a selective Janus kinase inhibitor approved for rheumatoid arthritis by the US Food and Drug Administration for the treatment of COVID-19, is a drug with both antiviral and anti-inflammatory properties. Decreased plasma IL-6, IL-1β, and TNF-α levels, rapid recovery of circulating T and B cells, and increased antibody development against SARS-CoV-2 virus spike protein have been reported in patients with severe COVID-19 treated with Janus kinase inhibitor [250].

COVID-19 who are intubated and do not respond to mechanical ventilation or pharmacological treatments with intensive care may be candidates for treatment with extracorporeal membrane oxygenation (ECMO). However, we need to know that ECMO applications negatively affect coagulation and inflammation.

Conclusion

We experienced a COVID-19 pandemic that affected the whole world in every sense, causing mass deaths, additional diseases, severe economic crises worldwide, and negatively affecting people's morale and motivation. Many studies have examined and tried to define the mechanisms of coagulopathy developing due to COVID-19 sepsis. However, the existing mechanisms have been insufficient to explain the coagulopathy that occurs. Unfortunately, the treatment strategies related to these did not give satisfactory results.

Although we did not leave it behind completely, we left the moderate and severe COVID-19 disease behind at the time I wrote the chapter. However, we may encounter different pandemics in the future. We must be prepared to eliminate such epidemics with the least damage. The most effective struggle is to take first-step measures such as hygiene and vaccination.

References

[1] Trzeciak, S, Zanotti-Cavazzoni, S, Parrillo, JE, Dellinger, RP. (2005). Inclusion criteria for clinical trials in sepsis: did the American College of Chest Physicians/ Society of Critical Care Medicine consensus conference definitions of sepsis have an impact? *Chest,* 127(1), 242-245.

[2] Welte T, Brunkhorst FM. 6th International Congress "Sepsis and Multiorgan Dysfunction"Weimar Sepsis Update 2013–Consensus and Controversies. *Infection.* 2013;41(1):S1-90.

[3] Kadri SS, Lai YL, Warner S, Strich JR, Babiker A, Ricotta EE, Demirkale CY, Dekker JP, Palmore TN, Rhee C, Klompas M. Inappropriate empirical antibiotic therapy for bloodstream infections based on discordant in-vitro susceptibilities: a retrospective cohort analysis of prevalence, predictors, and mortality risk in US hospitals. *The Lancet Infectious Diseases.* 2021 Feb 1;21(2):241-51.

[4] Angus DC, Linde-Zwirble WT, Lidicker J, Clermont G, Carcillo J, Pinsky MR. Epidemiology of severe sepsis in the United States: analysis of incidence, outcome, and associated costs of care. *Critical care medicine.* 2001 Jul 1;29(7):1303-10.

[5] Alberti C, Brun-Buisson C, Burchardi H, Martin C, Goodman S, Artigas A, Sicignano A, Palazzo M, Moreno R, Boulmé R, Lepage E. Epidemiology of sepsis and infection in ICU patients from an international multicentre cohort study. *Intensive care medicine.* 2002 Feb;28:108-21.

[6] Levy MM, Evans LE, Rhodes A. The surviving sepsis campaign bundle: 2018 update. *Intensive care medicine.* 2018 Jun;44:925-8.

[7] Li H, Liu L, Zhang D, Xu J, Dai H, Tang N, Su X, Cao B. SARS-CoV-2 and viral sepsis: observations and hypotheses. *The Lancet.* 2020 May 9;395(10235):1517-20.

[8] Singer M, Deutschman CS, Seymour CW, Shankar-Hari M, Annane D, Bauer M, Bellomo R, Bernard GR, Chiche JD, Coopersmith CM, Hotchkiss RS. The third international consensus definitions for sepsis and septic shock (Sepsis-3). *JAMA.* 2016 Feb 23;315(8):801-10.

[9] Vincent JL, Rello J, Marshall J, Silva E, Anzueto A, Martin CD, Moreno R, Lipman J, Gomersall C, Sakr Y, Reinhart K. International study of the prevalence and outcomes of infection in intensive care units. *JAMA.* 2009 Dec 2;302(21):2323-9.

[10] Rosendaal FR. Venous thrombosis: a multicausal disease. *The Lancet.* 1999 Apr 3;353(9159):1167-73.

[11] Esmon CT, Fukudome K, Mather T, Bode W, Regan LM, Stearns-Kurosawa DJ, Kurosawa S. Inflammation, sepsis, and coagulation. *Haematologica.* 1999 Jan 1;84(3):254-9.

[12] Foley JH, Conway EM. Cross talk pathways between coagulation and inflammation. *Circulation research.* 2016 Apr 29;118(9):1392-408.

[13] D'Elia RV, Harrison K, Oyston PC, Lukaszewski RA, Clark GC. Targeting the "cytokine storm" for therapeutic benefit. *Clinical and Vaccine Immunology.* 2013 Mar;20(3):319-27.

[14] Aird WC. "The role of the endothelium in severe sepsis and multiple organ dysfunction syndrome." *Blood.* 2003;101(10):3765–3777.

[15] Matsuda N. "Alert cell strategy in SIRS-induced vasculitis: sepsis and endothelial cells." *J. Intensive Care.* 2016;4:21.

[16] Ince C, Mayeux PR, Nguyen T, Gomez H, Kellum JA, Ospina-Tascón GA, Hernandez G, Murray P, De Backer D. The endothelium in sepsis. *Shock* (Augusta, Ga.). 2016 Mar;45(3):259.

[17] Hattori Y, Hattori K, Suzuki T, Matsuda N. "Recent advances in the pathophysiology and molecular basis of sepsis-associated organ dysfunction: Novel therapeutic implications and challenges." *Pharmacol. Ther.* 2017;177:56-66.

[18] Ahmad F, Kannan M, Ansari AW. Role of SARS-CoV-2-induced cytokines and growth factors in coagulopathy and thromboembolism. *Cytokine & Growth Factor Reviews.* 2022 Feb 1;63:58-68.

[19] Herter JM, Rossaint J, Zarbock A. Platelets in inflammation and immunity. *Journal of Thrombosis and Haemostasis.* 2014 Nov 1;12(11):1764-75.

[20] Chen Y, Zhong H, Zhao Y, Luo X, Gao W. Role of platelet biomarkers in inflammatory response. *Biomarker Research.* 2020 Dec;8:1-7.

[21] Levi M, Scully M. "How I treat disseminated intravascular coagulation." *Blood.* 2018;131(8):845–854.

[22] Liu Y, Gao W, Guo W, Guo Y, Shi M, Dong G, Ge Q, Zhu J, Lu J. Prominent coagulation disorder is closely related to inflammatory response and could be as a prognostic indicator for ICU patients with COVID-19. *Journal of thrombosis and thrombolysis.* 2020 Nov;50:825-32.

[23] Levi M, Van Der Poll T. "Inflammation and coagulation." *Crit. Care Med.* 2010;38(2 Suppl):S26–S34.

[24] Us D. "Cytokine storm in avian influenza." *Find Microbiome.* 2008;42(2):365-80.

[25] Jose RJ, Manuel A. "COVID-19 cytokine storm: the interplay between inflammation and coagulation." *Lancet Respir Med.* 2020; 8 (6):e46–e47.

[26] Liu Y, Yang Y, Zhang C, Huang F, Wang F, Yuan J, Wang Z, Li J, Li J, Feng C, Zhang Z. Clinical and biochemical indexes from 2019-nCoV infected patients

linked to viral loads and lung injury. *Science China Life Sciences*. 2020 Mar; 63:364-74.

[27] Mehta P, McAuley DF, Brown M, Sanchez E, Tattersall RS, Manson JJ. COVID-19: consider cytokine storm syndromes and immunosuppression. *The lancet.* 2020 Mar 28;395(10229):1033-4.

[28] Fajgenbaum DC, June CH "Cytokine storm." *N. Engl. J. Med.* 2020;383(23):2255–2273.

[29] Kaya Y. "Pathophysiology of Sepsis." *Journal of Intensive Care* 2005;5(2):80-84/.

[30] Magro C, Mulvey JJ, Berlin D, Nuovo G, Salvatore S, Harp J, Baxter-Stoltzfus A, Laurence J. Complement associated microvascular injury and thrombosis in the pathogenesis of severe COVID-19 infection: a report of five cases. *Translational Research.* 2020 Jun 1;220:1-3.

[31] Gupta S, Sakhuja A, Kumar G, McGrath E, Nanchal RS, Kashani KB. Culture-negative severe sepsis: nationwide trends and outcomes. *Chest.* 2016 Dec 1;150(6):1251-9.

[32] Engelmann B, Massberg S. "Thrombosis as an intravascular effector of innate immunity." *Nat Rev Immunol.* 2013; 13(1) :34–45.

[33] Rudd KE, Johnson SC, Agesa KM, Shackelford KA, Tsoi D, Kievlan DR, Colombara DV, Ikuta KS, Kissoon N, Finfer S, Fleischmann-Struzek C. Global, regional, and national sepsis incidence and mortality, 1990–2017: analysis for the Global Burden of Disease Study. *The Lancet.* 2020 Jan 18;395(10219):200-211.

[34] Schmidt K, Gensichen J, Fleischmann-Struzek C, Bahr V, Pausch C, Sakr Y, Reinhart K, Vollmar HC, Thiel P, Scherag A, Gantner J. Long-Term Survival Following Sepsis: Results of a Single-Center Registry Study With 4-Year Follow-Up. *Deutsches Ärzteblatt International.* 2020 Nov;117(46):775.

[35] Prescott HC, Osterholzer JJ, Langa KM, Angus DC, Iwashyna TJ. Late mortality after sepsis: propensity matched cohort study. *BMJ.* 2016 May 17;353.

[36] Esper AM, Martin GS. "Expanding the international epidemiology of sepsis: the impact of organ dysfunction." *Critical Care* 2009; 13:120.

[37] Danai P, Martin GS. "Sepsis epidemiology: recent developments." *Curr Infect Dis Rep* 2005; 7:3029.

[38] Martin GS, Mannino DM, Eaton S, Moss M. "The epidemiology of sepsis in the United States from 1979 through 2000." *N Engl J Med* 2003; 348:1546.

[39] Kaukonen KM, Bailey M, Suzuki S, Pilcher D, Bellomo R. Mortality related to severe sepsis and septic shock among critically ill patients in Australia and New Zealand, 2000-2012. *JAMA.* 2014 Apr 2;311(13):1308-1316.

[40] Angus DC, Kelley MA, Schmitz RJ. Current and projected workforce requirements for care. *JAMA.* 2000;284(21):2762-2770.

[41] Stevenson EK, Rubenstein AR, Radin GT, Wiener RS, Walkey AJ. Two decades of mortality trends among patients with severe sepsis: a comparative meta-analysis. *Critical care medicine.* 2014 Mar;42(3):625.

[42] Shankar-Hari M, Phillips GS, Levy ML, Seymour CW, Liu VX, Deutschman CS, Angus DC, Rubenfeld GD, Singer M. Developing a new definition and assessing new clinical criteria for septic shock: for the Third International Consensus

Definitions for Sepsis and Septic Shock (Sepsis-3). *JAMA*. 2016 Feb 23;315(8): 775-787.

[43] Cárdenas-Turanzas M, Ensor J, Wakefield C, Zhang K, Wallace SK, Price KJ, Nates JL. Cross-validation of a sequential organ failure assessment score–based model to predict mortality in patients with cancer admitted to the intensive care unit. *Journal of critical care*. 2012 Dec 1;27(6):673-680.

[44] Ferreira FL, Bota DP, Bross A, Mélot C, Vincent JL. "Serial evaluation of the SOFA score to predict outcome in critically ill patients." *JAMA* 2001;286(14): 1754–8.

[45] Yang Z, Hu Q, Huang F, Xiong S, Sun Y. The prognostic value of the SOFA score in patients with COVID-19: A retrospective, observational study. *Medicine*. 2021 Aug 8;100(32).

[46] Seymour CW, Liu VX, Iwashyna TJ, Brunkhorst FM, Rea TD, Scherag A, Rubenfeld G, Kahn JM, Shankar-Hari M, Singer M, Deutschman CS. Assessment of clinical criteria for sepsis: for the Third International Consensus Definitions for Sepsis and Septic Shock (Sepsis-3). *JAMA*. 2016 Feb 23;315(8):762-774.

[47] Kostakis I, Smith GB, Prytherch D, Meredith P, Price C, Chauhan A, Mortlock A, Schmidt P, Spice C, Fox L, Fleming D. The performance of the National Early Warning Score and National Early Warning Score 2 in hospitalised patients infected by the severe acute respiratory syndrome coronavirus 2 (SARS-CoV-2). *Resuscitation*. 2021 Feb 1;159:150-157.

[48] Osuchowski MF, Winkler MS, Skirecki T, Cajander S, Shankar-Hari M, Lachmann G, Monneret G, Venet F, Bauer M, Brunkhorst FM, Weis S. The COVID-19 puzzle: deciphering pathophysiology and phenotypes of a new disease entity. *The Lancet Respiratory Medicine*. 2021 Jun 1;9(6):6226-42.

[49] Mulder MM, Brandts L, Brüggemann RA, Koelmann M, Streng AS, Olie RH, Gietema HA, Spronk HM, van der Horst IC, Sels JW, Wildberger JE. Serial markers of coagulation and inflammation and the occurrence of clinical pulmonary thromboembolism in mechanically ventilated patients with SARS-CoV-2 infection; the prospective Maastricht intensive care COVID cohort. *Thrombosis Journal*. 2021 Dec;19(1):1-2.

[50] Baykara N, Akalın H, Arslantaş MK, Hancı V, Çağlayan Ç, Kahveci F, Demirağ K, Baydemir C, Ünal N. Epidemiology of sepsis in intensive care units in Turkey: a multicenter, point-prevalence study. *Critical Care*. 2018 Dec;22(1):1-4.

[51] Marshall JC, Cook DJ, Christou NV, Bernard GR, Sprung CL, Sibbald WJ. Multiple organ dysfunction score: a reliable descriptor of a complex clinical outcome. *Critical care medicine*. 1995 Oct 1;23(10):1638-1652.

[52] Le Gall JR, Klar J, Lemeshow S, Saulnier F, Alberti C, Artigas A, Teres D. The Logistic Organ Dysfunction system: a new way to assess organ dysfunction in the intensive care unit. *JAMA*. 1996 Sep 11;276(10):802-810.

[53] Vincent JL, Moreno R, Takala J, Willatts S, De Mendonça A, Bruining H, Reinhart CK, Suter P, Thijs LG. *The SOFA (Sepsis-related Organ Failure Assessment) score to describe organ dysfunction/failure: On behalf of the Working Group on Sepsis-Related Problems of the European Society of Intensive Care Medicine* (see contributors to the project in the appendix). (1996): 707-710.

[54] Vincent JL, Bihari DJ, Suter PM, Bruining HA, White J, Nicolas-Chanoin MH, Wolff M, Spencer RC, Hemmer M. The prevalence of nosocomial infection in intensive care units in Europe: results of the European Prevalence of Infection in Intensive Care (EPIC) Study. *JAMA*. 1995 Aug 23;274(8):639-644.

[55] Martin GS, Mannino DM, Moss M. "The effect of age on the development and outcome of adult sepsis." *Crit Care Med* 2006; 34:15.

[56] Falagas ME, Kompoti M. "Obesity and infection." *Lancet Infect Dis* 2006; 6:438.

[57] Dremsizov T, Clermont G, Kellum JA, Kalassian KG, Fine MJ, Angus DC. Severe sepsis in community-acquired pneumonia: when does it happen, and do systemic inflammatory response syndrome criteria help predict course? *Chest.* 2006 Apr 1;129(4):968-978.

[58] Prescott HC, Dickson RP, Rogers MA, Langa KM, Iwashyna TJ. Hospitalization type and subsequent severe sepsis. *American journal of respiratory and critical care medicine.* 2015 Sep 1;192(5):581-588.

[59] Netea MG, Van der Meer JW. "Immunodeficiency and genetic defects of pattern-recognition receptors." *N Engl J Med* 2011; 364:60.

[60] Williams MD, Braun LA, Cooper LM, Johnston J, Weiss RV, Qualy RL, Linde-Zwirble W. Hospitalized cancer patients with severe sepsis: analysis of incidence, mortality, and associated costs of care. *Critical care.* 2004 Oct;8(5):1-8.

[61] Zhou F, Yu T, Du R, Fan G, Liu Y, Liu Z, Xiang J, Wang Y, Song B, Gu X, Guan L. Clinical course and risk factors for mortality of adult inpatients with COVID-19 in Wuhan, China: a retrospective cohort study. *The lancet.* 2020 Mar 28;395(10229):1054-62.

[62] Haktanir A, Seki T, Dilmaç B. Adaptation and evaluation of Turkish version of the fear of COVID-19 scale. *Death studies.* 2022 Mar 16;46(3):719-727.

[63] Aird WC. Endothelium and haemostasis. *Hämostaseologie.* 2015;35(01):11-16.

[64] Aird WC. "Phenotypic heterogeneity of the endothelium: structure, function, and mechanisms." *Circ Res.* 2007;100((2)): 158–173.

[65] Pons S, Arnaud M, Loiselle M, Arrii E, Azoulay E, Zafrani L. Immune consequences of endothelial cells' activation and dysfunction during sepsis. *Critical care clinics.* 2020 Apr 1;36(2):401-413.

[66] Jaffe EA. "Cell biology of endothelial cells." *Hum Pathol* 1987; 18:234.

[67] Klein T, Ling Z, Heimberg H, Madsen OD, Heller RS, Serup P. Nestin is expressed in vascular endothelial cells in the adult human pancreas. *Journal of Histochemistry & Cytochemistry.* 2003 Jun;51(6):697-706.

[68] Cagno V, Tseligka ED, Jones ST, Tapparel C "Heparan sulfate proteoglycans and viral attachment: true receptors or adaptation bias?" *Viruses* 11(7):596, 2019.

[69] Stencel-Baerenwald JE, Reiss K, Reiter DM, Stehle T, Dermody TS. The sweet spot: defining virus–sialic acid interactions. *Nature Reviews Microbiology.* 2014 Nov;12(11):739-49.

[70] Uchimido R, Schmidt EP, Shapiro NI "The glycocalyx: a novel diagnostic and therapeutic target in sepsis." *Crit Care* 23(1):16, 2019.

[71] Gross PL, Aird WC. "The endothelium and thrombosis." *Semin Thromb Hemost* 2000; 26:463.

[72] Wagner DD, Frenette PS. "The vessel wall and its interactions." *Blood* 2008; 111:5271.

[73] Ünüvar A. COVID-19 ve koagülopati. Sağlık Bilimlerinde İleri Araştırmalar Dergisi [COVID-19 and coagulopathy. *Journal of Advanced Studies in Health Sciences*]. 2020;3(S1):53-62.

[74] Levi M, Keller TT, Van Gorp E, Ten Cate H. Infection and inflammation and the coagulation system. *Cardiovascular research.* 2003 Oct 15;60(1):26-39.

[75] Levi M, Ten Cate H. Disseminated intravascular coagulation. *New England Journal of Medicine.* 1999 Aug 19;341(8):586-592.

[76] Tay MZ, Poh CM, Rénia L, MacAry PA, Ng LF. The trinity of COVID-19: immunity, inflammation and intervention. *Nature Reviews Immunology.* 2020 Jun;20(6):363-374.

[77] Mercuro NJ, Yen CF, Shim DJ, Maher TR, McCoy CM, Zimetbaum PJ, Gold HS. Risk of QT interval prolongation associated with use of hydroxychloroquine with or without concomitant azithromycin among hospitalized patients testing positive for coronavirus disease 2019 (COVID-19). *JAMA cardiology.* 2020 Sep 1;5(9):1036-1041.

[78] Chen Y, Guo Y, Pan Y, Zhao ZJ. "Structure analysis of the receptor binding of 2019- nCoV." *Biochem Biophys Res Commun.* 2020; 525(1):135–140.

[79] Varga Z, Flammer AJ, Steiger P, Haberecker M, Andermatt R, Zinkernagel AS, Mehra MR, Schuepbach RA, Ruschitzka F, Moch H. Endothelial cell infection and endotheliitis in COVID-19. *The Lancet.* 2020 May 2;395(10234):1417-8.

[80] Gheblawi M, Wang K, Viveiros A, Nguyen Q, Zhong JC, Turner AJ, Raizada MK, Grant MB, Oudit GY. Angiotensin-converting enzyme 2: SARS-CoV-2 receptor and regulator of the renin-angiotensin system: celebrating the 20th anniversary of the discovery of ACE2. *Circulation research.* 2020 May 8;126(10):1456-1474.

[81] Alnima T, Mulder MM, Van Bussel BC, Ten Cate H. COVID-19 coagulopathy: from pathogenesis to treatment. *Acta Haematologica.* 2022;145(3):282-296.

[82] Teuwen LA, Geldhof V, Pasut A, Carmeliet P. "COVID- 19: the vasculature unleashed." *Nat Rev Immunol* 2020; 20:389.

[83] Libby P, Lüscher T. "COVID-19 is, in the end, an endothelial disease." *Eur Heart J* 2020; 41:3038.

[84] Hadi HA, Carr CS, Al Suwaidi J. "Endothelial dysfunction: cardiovascular risk factors, therapy, and outcome. Vasc." *Health Risk Management.* 2005;1(3):183–198.

[85] Yau JW, Teoh H., Verma S. "Endothelial cell control of thrombosis." *BMC Cardiovasc. Discord.* 2015;15:130.

[86] Ciceri F, Beretta L, Scandroglio AM, Colombo S, Landoni G, Ruggeri A, Peccatori J, D'Angelo A, De Cobelli F, Rovere-Querini P, Tresoldi M. Microvascular COVID-19 lung vessels obstructive thromboinflammatory syndrome (MicroCLOTS): an atypical acute respiratory distress syndrome working hypothesis. *Critical care and resuscitation.* 2020 Jun;22(2):95-97.

[87] Hulshof AM, Brüggemann RA, Mulder MM, Van de Berg TW, Sels JW, Olie RH, Spaetgens B, Streng AS, Verhezen P, Van der Horst IC, Ten Cate H. Serial EXTEM, FIBTEM, and tPA rotational thromboelastometry observations in the

Maastricht Intensive Care COVID cohort—persistence of hypercoagulability and hypofibrinolysis despite anticoagulation. *Frontiers in cardiovascular medicine.* 2021 Apr 26;8:654174.

[88] Connors JM, Levy JH. "COVID-19 and its implications for thrombosis and anticaogulation." *Blood.* 2020;135(23):2033–2040.

[89] Iba T, Levy JH, Warkentin TE, Thachil J, Van Der Poll T, Levi M. Scientific and Standardization Committee on DIC, and the Scientific and Standardization Committee on Perioperative and Critical Care of the International Society on Thrombosis and Haemostasis. Diagnosis and management of sepsis-induced coagulopathy and disseminated intravascular coagulation. *J Thromb Haemost.* 2019 Nov;17(11):1989-1994.

[90] Gando S, Levi M, Toh CH. Disseminated intravascular coagulation. *Nature reviews Disease primers.* 2016 Jun 2;2(1):1-6.

[91] Heit JA, Silverstein MD, Mohr DN, Petterson TM, O'Fallon WM, Melton LJ. Predictors of survival after deep vein thrombosis and pulmonary embolism: a population-based, cohort study. *Archives of internal medicine.* 1999 Mar 8;159(5):445-453.

[92] Li JY, Wang HF, Yin P, Li D, Wang DL, Peng P, Wang WH, Wang L, Yuan XW, Xie JY, Zhou F. Clinical characteristics and risk factors for symptomatic venous thromboembolism in hospitalized COVID-19 patients: a multicenter retrospective study. *Journal of Thrombosis and Haemostasis.* 2021 Apr;19(4):1038-1048.

[93] Jenner WJ, Kanji R, Mirsadraee S, Gue YX, Price S, Prasad S, Gorog DA. Thrombotic complications in 2928 patients with COVID-19 treated in intensive care: a systematic review. *Journal of thrombosis and thrombolysis.* 2021 Apr;51:595-607.

[94] Le Jeune S, Suhl J, Benainous R, Minvielle F, Purser C, Foudi F, Warzocha U, Dhote R. High prevalence of early asymptomatic venous thromboembolism in anticoagulated COVID-19 patients hospitalized in general wards. *Journal of thrombosis and thrombolysis.* 2021 Apr;51:637-641.

[95] Zhang C, Shen L, Le KJ, Pan MM, Kong LC, Gu ZC, Xu H, Zhang Z, Ge WH, Lin HW. Incidence of venous thromboembolism in hospitalized coronavirus disease 2019 patients: a systematic review and meta-analysis. *Frontiers in Cardiovascular Medicine.* 2020 Aug 6;7:151.

[96] Klok FA, Kruip MJ, Van der Meer NJ, Arbous MS, Gommers DA, Kant KM, Kaptein FH, van Paassen J, Stals MA, Huisman MV, Endeman H. Incidence of thrombotic complications in critically ill ICU patients with COVID-19. *Thrombosis research.* 2020 Jul 1;191:145-147.

[97] Levi M, Thachil J, Iba T, Levy JH. Coagulation abnormalities and thrombosis in patients with COVID-19. *The Lancet Haematology.* 2020 Jun 1;7(6):e438-440.

[98] Munoz-Rivas N, Abad-Motos A, Mestre-Gomez B, Sierra-Hidalgo F, Cortina-Camarero C, Lorente-Ramos RM, Torres-Rubio P, Arranz-Garcia P, Franco-Moreno AI, Gomez-Mariscal E, Mauleon-Fernandez C. Systemic thrombosis in a large cohort of COVID-19 patients despite thromboprophylaxis: A retrospective study. *Thrombosis research.* 2021 Mar 1;199:132-142.

[99] Lodigiani C, Iapichino G, Carenzo L, Cecconi M, Ferrazzi P, Sebastian T, Kucher N, Studt JD, Sacco C, Bertuzzi A, Sandri MT. Venous and arterial thromboembolic complications in COVID-19 patients admitted to an academic hospital in Milan, Italy. *Thrombosis research.* 2020 Jul 1;191:9-14.

[100] Indes JE, Koleilat I, Hatch AN, Choinski K, Jones DB, Aldailami H, Billett H, Denesopolis JM, Lipsitz E. Early experience with arterial thromboembolic complications in patients with COVID-19. *Journal of vascular surgery.* 2021 Feb 1;73(2):381-9.

[101] Libby P, Simon DI. "Inflammation and thrombosis: the clot thickens." *Circulation,* 103 (13) (2001), pp. 1718-1720.

[102] Giamarellos-Bourboulis EJ, Netea MG, Rovina N, Akinosoglou K, Antoniadou A, Antonakos N, Damoraki G, Gkavogianni T, Adami ME, Katsaounou P, Ntaganou M. Complex immune dysregulation in COVID-19 patients with severe respiratory failure. *Cell host & microbe.* 2020 Jun 10;27(6):992-1000.

[103] Orfeo T, Butenas S, Brummel-Ziedins KE, Mann KG. "The tissue factor requirement in blood coagulation." *J Biol Chem.* 2005;280:42887-42896.

[104] Iba T, Levy JH. "Inflammation and thrombosis: roles of neutrophils, platelets, and endothelial cells and their interactions in thrombus formation during sepsis." *J Thromb Haemost.* 2018; 16 (2):231–241.

[105] Burzynski LC, Humphry M, Pyrillou K, Wiggins KA, Chan JN, Figg N, Kitt LL, Summers C, Tatham KC, Martin PB, Bennett MR. The coagulation and immune systems are directly linked through the activation of interleukin-1α by thrombin. *Immunity.* 2019 Apr 16;50(4):1033-1042.

[106] Thornton P, McColl BW, Greenhalgh A, Denes A, Allan SM, Rothwell NJ. Platelet interleukin-1α drives cerebrovascular inflammation. *Blood, The Journal of the American Society of Hematology.* 2010 Apr 29;115(17):3632-3639.

[107] Cavalli G, Colafrancesco S, Emmi G, Imazio M, Lopalco G, Maggio MC, Sota J, Dinarello CA. Interleukin 1α: a comprehensive review on the role of IL-1α in the pathogenesis and treatment of autoimmune and inflammatory diseases. *Autoimmunity reviews.* 2021 Mar 1;20(3):102763.

[108] Goshua G, Pine AB, Meizlish ML, Chang CH, Zhang H, Bahel P, Baluha A, Bar N, Bona RD, Burns AJ, Cruz CS. Endotheliopathy in COVID-19-associated coagulopathy: evidence from a single-centre, cross-sectional study. *The Lancet Haematology.* 2020 Aug 1;7(8):e575-82.

[109] Vischer UM "von Willebrand factor, endothelial dysfunction, and cardiovascular disease." *J. Thromb. haemost* 2006;4(6):1186–1193.

[110] Kawecki C, Lenting PJ, Denis CV, "von Willebrand factor and inflammation," *J. Thromb. haemost* 15 (7) (2017) 1285–1294.

[111] Bels JL, Van Kuijk SM, Ghossein-Doha C, Tijssen FH, Van Gassel RJ, Tas J, Schnabel RM, Aries MJ, van de Poll MC, Bergmans DC, Meex SJ. Decreased serial scores of severe organ failure assessments are associated with survival in mechanically ventilated patients; the prospective Maastricht Intensive Care COVID cohort. *Journal of Critical Care.* 2021 Apr 1;62:38-45.

[112] Jones SA, Hunter CA "Is IL-6 a key cytokine target for therapy in COVID-19?" *Nat. Rev. Immunol.* 2021;21(6):337–339.

[113] Perrone LA Plowden JK, García-Sastre A, Katz JM, Tumpey TM. "H5N1 and 1918 pandemic influenza virus infection results in early and excessive infiltration of macrophages and neutrophils in the lungs of mice." *PLoS Pathog.* 2008;4(8):e1000115.
[114] Hattori Y, Takano KI, Teramae H, Yamamoto S, Yokoo H, Matsuda N. Insights into sepsis therapeutic design based on the apoptotic death pathway. *Journal of pharmacological sciences.* 2010;114(4):354-365.
[115] Hotchkiss RS, Tinsley KW, Swanson PE, Karl IE. "Endothelial cell apoptosis in sepsis." *Crit. Care Med.* 2002;30(Supplement):S225–S228.
[116] Bannerman DD, Goldblum SE. "Mechanisms of bacterial lipopolysaccharide-induced endothelial apoptosis." *Am. J. Physiol. Lung Cell. Mol. Physiol.* 2003;284 (6):L899–L914.
[117] Zhou M. Simms HH, Wang P. "Adrenomedullin and adrenomedullin binding protein-1 attenuate vascular endothelial cell apoptosis in sepsis." *Ann. Surg.* 2004;240(2):321–330.
[118] Hutchins NA, Chung CS, Borgerding JN, Ayala CA., Ayala A. Kupffer cells protect liver sinusoidal endothelial cells from Fas-dependent apoptosis in sepsis by down-regulating gp130. *The American journal of pathology.* 2013 Mar 1;182(3): 742-754.
[119] Gill SE, Rohan M, Mehta S. "Role of pulmonary microvascular endothelial cell apoptosis in murine sepsis-induced lung injury in vivo." *Repir. Res.* 2015;16(1): 109.
[120] Meyrick B. "Pathology of the adult respiratory distress syndrome." *Crit. Care Clin.* 1986;2(3):405–428.
[121] Helms, J, Kremer, S, Merdji, H, Clere-Jehl, R, Schenck, M, Kummerlen, C, Meziani, F. (2020). Neurologic features in severe SARS-CoV-2 infection. *New England Journal of Medicine,* 382(23), 2268-2270.
[122] Oxley, T, Mocco, J, Majidi, S. Large-vessel stroke as a presenting feature of Covid-19 in the young [2020]. *NEJM* doi, 10.
[123] Xu, Z, Shi, L, Wang, Y, Zhang, J, Huang, L, Zhang, C, Wang, FS. (2020). Pathological findings of COVID-19 associated with acute respiratory distress syndrome. *The Lancet respiratory medicine,* 8(4), 420-422.
[124] Kirschenbaum, D, Imbach, LL, Rushing, EJ, Frauenknecht, KB, Gascho, D, Ineichen, BV, Frontzek, K. (2021). Intracerebral endotheliitis and microbleeds are neuropathological features of COVID-19. *Neuropathology and applied neurobiology,* 47(3), 454-459.
[125] Campbell, RA, Hisada, Y, Denorme, F, Grover, SP, Bouck, EG, Middleton, EA, Mackman, N. (2021). Comparison of the coagulopathies associated with COVID-19 and sepsis. *Research and practice in thrombosis and haemostasis,* 5(4), e12525.
[126] Blot, M, de Maistre, E, Bourredjem, A, Quenot, JP, Nguyen, M, Bouhemad, B., Piroth, L. (2021). Specific features of the coagulopathy signature in severe COVID-19 pneumonia. *Frontiers in Medicine,* 8, 675191.
[127] Han, H, Yang, L, Liu, R, Liu, F, Wu, KL, Li, J, Zhu, CL. (2020). Prominent changes in blood coagulation of patients with SARS-CoV-2 infection. *Clinical Chemistry and Laboratory Medicine* (CCLM), 58(7), 1116-1120.

[128] Busch, MH, Timmermans, SA, Nagy, M, Visser, M, Huckriede, J, Aendekerk, JP, Van Paassen, P. (2020). Neutrophils and contact activation of coagulation as potential drivers of COVID-19. *Circulation,* 142(18), 1787-1790.

[129] Du, X, Liu, H, Yue, Y, Wu, Q, Jiang, W, Qiu, Y, Zeng, Y. (2021). Anisodamine hydrobromide protects glycocalyx and against the lipopolysaccharide-induced increases in microvascular endothelial layer permeability and nitric oxide production. *Cardiovascular engineering and technology,* 12, 91-100.

[130] Choudhary S, Sharma K, Singh H, Silakari O. "The interplay between inflammatory pathways and COVID-19: a critical review on pathogenesis and therapeutic options." *Microbe Pathog.* 2021; 150:104673.

[131] Zhou, F, Yu, T, Du, R, Fan, G, Liu, Y, Liu, Z, Cao, B. (2020). Clinical course and risk factors for mortality of adult inpatients with COVID-19 in Wuhan, China: a retrospective cohort study. *The lancet,* 395(10229), 1054-1062.

[132] Zhang, C, Wu, Z, Li, JW, Zhao, H, Wang, GQ. (2020). Cytokine release syndrome in severe COVID-19: interleukin-6 receptor antagonist tocilizumab may be the key to reduce mortality. *International journal of antimicrobial agents,* 55(5), 105954.

[133] Tang, J, Lin, J, Zhang, E., Zhong, M, Luo, Y, Fu, Y, Yang, Y. (2021). Serum IL-6 and procalcitonin are two promising novel biomarkers for evaluating the severity of COVID-19 patients. *Medicine,* 100(22).

[134] Magunia, H, Lederer, S, Verbuecheln, R, Gilot, BJ, Koeppen, M., Haeberle, HA, Rosenberger, P. (2021). Machine learning identifies ICU outcome predictors in a multicenter COVID-19 cohort. *Critical Care*, 25, 1-14.

[135] Burstein SA. "Cytokines, platelet productions and hemostasis." *Platelets.* 1997;8:93-104.

[136] Taylor, FB, Chang, A, Esmon, CT, D'angelo, A, Vigano-D'Angelo, S, Blick, KE. (1987). Protein C prevents the coagulopathic and lethal effects of Escherichia coli infusion in the baboon. *The Journal of clinical investigation,* 79(3), 918-925.

[137] Wang J, Jiang M, Chen X, Montaner LJ "Cytokine storm and leukocyte changes in mild versus severe SARS-CoV-2 infection: Review of 3939 COVID-19 patients in China and emerging pathogenesis and therapy concepts." *J. Leukoc. biol.* 2020; 108 (1):17–41.

[138] Kang S, Kishimoto T. "Interplay between interleukin-6 signaling and the vascular endothelium in cytokine storms." *Exp. Mole. Med.* 2021; 53 (7):1116–1123.

[139] Brosnahan, SB, Smilowitz, NR, Amoroso, NE, Barfield, M, Berger, JS, Goldenberg, R, Maldonado, TS. (2021). Thrombosis at hospital presentation in patients with and without coronavirus disease 2019. *Journal of Vascular Surgery: Venous and Lymphatic Disorders,* 9(4), 845-852.

[140] Wang, G, Wu, C, Zhang, Q, Wu, F, Yu, B, Lv, J, Zhong, Y. (2020, May). C-reactive protein level may predict the risk of COVID-19 aggravation. In *Open forum infectious diseases* (Vol. 7, No. 5, p. 153). US: Oxford University Press.

[141] Bozzani, A, Arici, V, Tavazzi, G., Franciscone, MM, Danesino, V, Rota, M, Ragni, F. (2020). Acute arterial and deep venous thromboembolism in COVID-19 patients: risk factors and personalized therapy. *Surgery,* 168(6), 987-992.

[142] Xu, JB, Xu, C, Zhang, RB, Wu, M, Pan, CK, Li, XJ, Zhu, S. (2020). Associations of procalcitonin, C-reaction protein and neutrophil-to-lymphocyte ratio with

mortality in hospitalized COVID-19 patients in China. *Scientific reports,* 10(1), 1-10.

[143] Huang, C, Wang, Y, Li, X, Ren, L, Zhao, J, Hu, Y, Cao, B. (2020). Clinical features of patients infected with 2019 novel coronavirus in Wuhan, China. *The lancet,* 395(10223), 497-506.

[144] Najem MY, Couturaud F, Lemarie CA "Cytokine and chemokine regulation of venous thromboembolism." *J. Thromb. Haemost.,* 18 (5) (2020), pp. 1009-1019.

[145] Demetz G, Ott I "The interface between inflammation and coagulation in cardiovascular disease." *Int. J. Inflam.*, 2012, Article 860301.

[146] Perreau, M, Suffiotti, M, Marques-Vidal, P, Wiedemann, A, Levy, Y, Laouénan, C, Pantaleo, G. (2021). The cytokines HGF and CXCL13 predict the severity and the mortality in COVID-19 patients. *Nature Communications,* 12(1), 4888.

[147] Herbert JM, Savi P, Laplace MC, Lale A "IL-4 inhibitors LPS-, IL-1 beta- and TNF alpha-induced expression of tissue factor in endothelial cells and monocytes." *FEBS Lett.,* 310 (1) (1992), pp. 31-33.

[148] Van Hinsbergh VW, Van den Berg EA, Fiers W, Dooijewaard G"Tumor necrosis factor induces the production of urokinase-type plasminogen activator by human endothelial cells." *Blood,* 75 (10) (1990), pp. 1991-1998.

[149] Godier, A, Clausse, D, Meslin, S, Bazine, M, Lang, E., Huche, F, Hamada, SR (2021). Major bleeding complications in critically ill patients with COVID-19 pneumonia. *Journal of thrombosis and thrombolysis,* 52, 18-21.

[150] Whyte, CS, Morrow, GB, Mitchell, JL, Chowdary, P, Mutch, NJ. (2020). Fibrinolytic abnormalities in acute respiratory distress syndrome (ARDS) and versatility of thrombolytic drugs to treat COVID-19. *Journal of Thrombosis and Haemostasis,* 18(7), 1548-1555.

[151] Liao, D, Zhou, F, Luo, L, Xu, M, Wang, H, Xia, J, Hu, Y. (2020). Haematological characteristics and risk factors in the classification and prognosis evaluation of COVID-19: a retrospective cohort study. *The Lancet Haematology,* 7(9), e671-e678.

[152] Levi M, Ten Cate H, Van der Poll T. "Endothelium: interface between coagulation and inflammation." *Critcare Med.* 2002; 30 ((5 Suppl l)):S220–4.

[153] Giesen, PL, Rauch, U, Bohrmann, B, Kling, D, Roqué, M., Fallon, JT, Nemerson, Y. (1999). Blood-borne tissue factor: another view of thrombosis. *Proceedings of the National Academy of Sciences,* 96(5), 2311-2315.

[154] Henn, V, Slupsky, JR, Gräfe, M, Anagnostopoulos, I, Förster, R, Müller-Berghaus, G, Kroczek, RA. (1998). CD40 ligand on activated platelets triggers an inflammatory reaction of endothelial cells. *Nature,* 391(6667), 591-594.

[155] Huang I, Pranata R. "Lymphopenia in severe coronavirus disease-2019 (COVID-19): systematic review and meta-analysis." *J Intensive Care.* 2020;8(1):36.

[156] Mao, J, Dai, R, Du, RC, Zhu, Y, Shui, LP, Luo, XH. (2021). Hematologic changes predict clinical outcome in recovered patients with COVID-19. *Annals of hematology,* 100, 675-689.

[157] Zhao, Q, Meng, M, Kumar, R, Wu, Y, Huang, J, Deng, Y, Yang, L. (2020). Lymphopenia is associated with severe coronavirus disease 2019 (COVID-19)

infections: A systemic review and meta-analysis. *International journal of infectious diseases,* 96, 131-135.

[158] Vinayagam S, Sattu K. "SARS-CoV-2 and coagulation disorders in diferent organs." *Life Sci.* 2020;260:118431.

[159] Qu, R, Ling, Y, Zhang, YHZ, Wei, LY, Chen, X, Li, XM, Wang, Q. (2020). Platelet-to-lymphocyte ratio is associated with prognosis in patients with coronavirus disease-19. *Journal of medical virology,* 92(9), 1533-1541.

[160] Zong, X, Gu, Y, Yu, H, Li, Z, Wang, Y. (2021). Thrombocytopenia is associated with COVID-19 severity and outcome: an updated meta-analysis of 5637 patients with multiple outcomes. *Laboratory Medicine,* 52(1), 10-15.

[161] Yang, X, Yang, Q, Wang, Y, Wu, Y, Xu, J, Yu, Y, Shang, Y. (2020). Thrombocytopenia and its association with mortality in patients with COVID-19. *Journal of Thrombosis and Haemostasis,* 18(6), 1469-1472.

[162] Yang AP, Liu J, Tao W, Li HM. "The diagnostic and predictive role of NLR, d-NLR and PLR in COVID-19 patients." *Int Immunopharmacol.* 2020;84:106504.

[163] Liu, Y, Du, X, Chen, J, Jin, Y, Peng, L, Wang, HH, Zhao, Y. (2020). Neutrophil-to-lymphocyte ratio as an independent risk factor for mortality in hospitalized patients with COVID-19. *Journal of Infection,* 81(1), e6-e12.

[164] Papayannopoulos V, Zychlinsky A. "NETs: a new strategy for using old weapons." *Trends Immunol* 2009; 30: 513-21.

[165] Mesa MA, Vasquez G. "NETosis." *Autoimmun Dis* 2013; 1:1-7.

[166] Kumar V, Sharma A. "Neutrophils: cinderella of innate immune system." *Int Immunopharmacol* 2010; 10: 1325-34.

[167] Gillot, C, Favresse, J, Mullier, F, Lecompte, T, Dogne, JM, Douxfils, J. (2021). NETosis and the immune system in COVID-19: mechanisms and potential treatments. *Frontiers in pharmacology,* 12, 708302.

[168] Brinkmann, V, Reichard, U, Goosmann, C, Fauler, B, Uhlemann, Y, Weiss, DS, Zychlinsky, A. (2004). Neutrophil extracellular traps kill bacteria. *Science,* 303(5663), 1532-1535.

[169] Tanaka, K, Koike, Y, Shimura, T, Okigami, M, Ide, S, Toiyama, Y, Kusunoki, M. (2014). In vivo characterization of neutrophil extracellular traps in various organs of a murine sepsis model. *PloS one,* 9(11), e111888.

[170] Kolaczkowska, E, Jenne, C.N, Surewaard, BG, Thanabalasuriar, A, Lee, WY, Sanz, MJ, Kubes, P. (2015). Molecular mechanisms of NET formation and degradation revealed by intravital imaging in the liver vasculature. *Nature communications,* 6(1), 6673.

[171] Manne, BK, Denorme, F, Middleton, EA, Portier, I, Rowley, JW, Stubben, C, Campbell, RA. (2020). Platelet gene expression and function in patients with COVID-19. *Blood,* 136(11), 1317-1329.

[172] Manda A, Pruchniak MP, Arazna M, Demkow UA. "Neutrophil extracellular traps in physiology and pathology." *Cent EJ Immunol* 2014; 39: 116-21.

[173] Zhang, D, Chen, G, Manwani, D, Mortha, A, Xu, C, Faith, JJ, Frenette, PS. (2015). Neutrophil ageing is regulated by the microbiome. *Nature,* 525(7570), 528-532.

[174] Fuchs, TA, Brill, A, Duerschmied, D, Schatzberg, D, Monestier, M, Myers Jr, D. D, Wagner, DD. (2010). Extracellular DNA traps promote thrombosis. *Proceedings of the National Academy of Sciences,* 107(36), 15880-15885.

[175] Martinod K, Wagner DD. "Thrombosis: tangled up in NETs." *Blood* 2014; 123:2768.

[176] Martinod, K, Demers, M, Fuchs, TA, Wong, SL, Brill, A, Gallant, M, Wagner, DD. (2013). Neutrophil histone modification by peptidylarginine deiminase 4 is critical for deep vein thrombosis in mice. *Proceedings of the National Academy of Sciences,* 110(21), 8674-8679.

[177] Martinod, K., Fuchs, TA, Zitomersky, NL, Wong, SL, Demers, M, Gallant, M, Wagner, DD. (2015). PAD4-deficiency does not affect bacteremia in polymicrobial sepsis and ameliorates endotoxemic shock. *Blood, The Journal of the American Society of Hematology,* 125(12), 1948-1956.

[178] Sollberger G, Tilley DO, Zychlinsky A. "Neutrophil extracellular traps: the biology of chromatin externalization." *Giant Cell.* 2018;44((5)):542–53.

[179] Noubouossie, DF, Whelihan, MF, Yu, YB, Sparkenbaugh, E, Pawlinski, R, Monroe, DM, Key, NS. (2017). In vitro activation of coagulation by human neutrophil DNA and histone proteins but not neutrophil extracellular traps. *Blood, The Journal of the American Society of Hematology,* 129(8), 1021-1029.

[180] McDonald, B, Davis, RP, Kim, SJ, Tse, M, Esmon, CT, Kolaczkowska, E, Jenne, CN. (2017). Platelets and neutrophil extracellular traps collaborate to promote intravascular coagulation during sepsis in mice. *Blood, The Journal of the American Society of Hematology,* 129(10), 1357-1367.

[181] Chen, J, Fu, X, Wang, Y, Ling, M, McMullen, B., Kulman, J, López, JA. (2010). Oxidative modification of von Willebrand factor by neutrophil oxidants inhibits its cleavage by ADAMTS13. *Blood, The Journal of the American Society of Hematology,* 115(3), 706-712.

[182] Papayannopoulos V, Metzler KD, Hakkim A, Zychlinsky A. "Neutrophil elastase and myeloperoxidase regulate the formation of neutrophil extracellular traps." *J Cell Biol.* 2010;191(3):677–691.

[183] Zhou, P, Yang, XL, Wang, XG, Hu, B, Zhang, L, Zhang, W, Shi, ZL. (2020). A pneumonia outbreak associated with a new coronavirus of probable bat origin. *Nature,* 579(7798), 270-273.

[184] Santiesteban-Lores LE, Cabrera-Crespo J, Carvalho E. "A double edged-sword: the complement system during SARS-CoV-2 infection." *Life Sci.* 2021;272:119245.

[185] Visser M, Heitmeier S, Ten Cate H, Spronk HMH. "Role of factor XIa and plasma kallikrein in arterial and venous thrombosis." *Thromb Haemost.* 2020;120((6)):883–993.

[186] Ackermann, M, Verleden, SE, Kuehnel, M, Haverich, A, Welte, T, Laenger, F, Jonigk, D. (2020). Pulmonary vascular endothelialitis, thrombosis, and angiogenesis in Covid-19. *New England Journal of Medicine,* 383(2), 120-128.

[187] Fox, SE, Akmatbekov, A, Harbert, JL, Li, G, Brown, JQ, Vander Heide, RS. (2020). Pulmonary and cardiac pathology in African American patients with COVID-19: an autopsy series from New Orleans. *The Lancet Respiratory Medicine,* 8(7), 681-686.

[188] Lax, SF, Skok, K, Zechner, P, Kessler, HH, Kaufmann, N, Koelblinger, C, Trauner, M. (2020). Pulmonary arterial thrombosis in COVID-19 with fatal outcome: results from a prospective, single-center, clinicopathologic case series. *Annals of internal medicine,* 173(5), 350-361.
[189] Middeldorp, S, Coppens, M, Van Haaps, TF, Foppen, M, Vlaar, AP, Müller, MC, Van Es, N. (2020). Incidence of venous thromboembolism in hospitalized patients with COVID-19. *Journal of Thrombosis and Haemostasis,* 18(8), 1995-2002.
[190] Du, Y, Tu, L, Zhu, P, Mu, M, Wang, R, Yang, P, Xu, G. (2020). Clinical features of 85 fatal cases of COVID-19 from Wuhan. A retrospective observational study. *American journal of respiratory and critical care medicine,* 201(11), 1372-1379.
[191] Zhang T, Sun LX, Feng RE. "Comparison of clinical and pathological features between severe acute respiratory syndrome and coronavirus disease 2019." *Zhonghua Jie He He Hu Xi Za Zhi.* 2020; 43 (6):496–502.
[192] Bonaventura, A, Vecchié, A, Dagna, L, Martinod, K, Dixon, DL, Van Tassell, BW, Abbate, A. (2021). Endothelial dysfunction and immunothrombosis as key pathogenic mechanisms in COVID-19. *Nature Reviews Immunology,* 21(5), 319-329.
[193] Andre, P, Prasad, KS, Denis, CV, He, M, Papalia, JM, Hynes, RO, Wagner, DD. (2002). CD40L stabilizes arterial thrombi by a β3 integrin–dependent mechanism. *Nature medicine,* 8(3), 247-252.
[194] Scudiero, F, Silverio, A, Di Maio, M, Russo, V, Citro, R, Personeni, D, Network, CI. (2021). Pulmonary embolism in COVID-19 patients: prevalence, predictors and clinical outcome. *Thrombosis research,* 198, 34-39.
[195] Peiró, AM, Gasch, AG, Bosch, MM. (2017). Update on the risk stratification of acute symptomatic pulmonary thromboembolism. *Revista Clínica Española* (English Edition), 217(6), 342-350.
[196] Miró, Ò, Jiménez, S, Llorens, P, Roussel, M, Gorlicki, J, García-Lamberechts, E. J, Freund, Y. (2022). Pulmonary embolism severity and in-hospital mortality: an international comparative study between COVID-19 and non-COVID patients. *European Journal of Internal Medicine,* 98, 69-76.
[197] Elsoukkary, SS, Mostyka, M, Dillard, A, Berman, DR, Ma, LX, Chadburn, A., Salvatore, SP. (2021). Autopsy findings in 32 patients with COVID-19: a single-institution experience. *Pathobiology,* 88(1), 56-68.
[198] Colling ME, Tourdot BE, Kanthi Y. "Inflammation, infection and venous thromboembolism." *Circ Res.* 2021; 128 ((12)):2017–36.
[199] Nevzorova, TA, Mordakhanova, ER, Daminova, AG, Ponomareva, AA, Andrianova, IA, Le Minh, G, Weisel, JW. (2019). Platelet factor 4-containing immune complexes induce platelet activation followed by calpain-dependent platelet death. *Cell death discovery,* 5(1), 106.
[200] Zhu W, Schrottmaier WC, Salzmann M, Rayes J. "SARS-CoV-2 receptor binding domain-specific antibodies activate platelets with features resembling the pathogenic antibodies in heparin-induced thrombocytopenia." *Res Sq.* 2021.
[201] Assinger A, Schrottmaier WC, Salzmann M, Rayes J. "Platelets in sepsis: an update on experimental models and clinical data." *Front Immunol.* 2019;10:1687.

[202] Aleem, A, Nadeem, AJ. (2022). *Coronavirus (COVID-19) vaccine-induced immune thrombotic thrombocytopenia (VITT).* StatPearls.

[203] Greinacher, A, Thiele, T, Warkentin, TE, Weisser, K, Kyrle, PA, Eichinger, S. (2021). Thrombotic thrombocytopenia after ChAdOx1 nCov-19 vaccination. *New England Journal of Medicine,* 384(22), 2092-2101.

[204] Nicholls, JM, Poon, LL, Lee, KC, Ng, WF, Lai, ST, Leung, CY, Peiris, JM. (2003). Lung pathology of fatal severe acute respiratory syndrome. *The Lancet,* 361(9371), 1773-1778.

[205] Satış, H, Özger, HS, Yıldız, PA, Hızel, K, Gulbahar, Ö, Erbaş, G, Tufan, A. (2021). Prognostic value of interleukin-18 and its association with other inflammatory markers and disease severity in COVID-19. *Cytokine,* 137, 155302.

[206] Soy M, Atagündüz P, Atagündüz I, Sucak GT. "Hemophagocytic lymphohistiocytosis: a review inspired by the COVID-19 pandemic." *Rheumatology International* 2021; 41(1):7-18.

[207] Zehnder, JL, Leung, LL, Landaw, SA. (2008). *Clinical use of coagulation tests.* Waltham, MA: UpToDate.

[208] Hirsh J, Poller L. "The international normalized ratio. A guide to understanding and correcting its problems." *Arch Intern Med,* 154 (1994), pp. 282-288.

[209] Iba T, Levy JH, Levi M, Thachil J. "Coagulopathy in COVID-19." *J Thromb Haemostasis,* 18 (2020), pp. 2103-2109.

[210] Bikdeli, B, Madhavan, MV, Jimenez, D, Chuich, T, Dreyfus, I, Driggin, E, Lip, GY. (2020). COVID-19 and thrombotic or thromboembolic disease: implications for prevention, antithrombotic therapy, and follow-up: JACC state-of-the-art review. *Journal of the American college of cardiology,* 75(23), 2950-2973.

[211] Cannegieter SC, Klok FA. "COVID-19 associated coagulopathy and thromboembolic disease: Commentary on an interim expert guidance." *Res Pract Thromb Haemost* 2020 April 20.

[212] Zhou, F, Yu, T, Du, R, Fan, G, Liu, Y, Liu, Z, Cao, B. (2020). Clinical course and risk factors for mortality of adult inpatients with COVID-19 in Wuhan, China: a retrospective cohort study. *The lancet,* 395(10229), 1054-1062.

[213] Thachil, J, Tang, N, Gando, S, Falanga, A, Levi, M, Clark, C, Iba, T. (2020). Laboratory haemostasis monitoring in COVID-19. *Journal of Thrombosis and Haemostasis,* 18(8), 2058.

[214] Thachil J. "What do monitoring platelet counts in COVID-19 teach us?" *J Thromb Haemost* 2020 Apr 28. doi: 10.1111/jth.14879.

[215] Thachil, J, Tang, N, Gando, S, Falanga, A, Cattaneo, M, Levi, M, Iba, T. (2020). ISTH interim guidance on recognition and management of coagulopathy in COVID-19. *Journal of Thrombosis and Haemostasis,* 18(5), 1023-1026.

[216] Li, X, Xu, S, Yu, M, Wang, K, Tao, Y, Zhou, Y, Zhao, J. (2020). Risk factors for severity and mortality in adult COVID-19 inpatients in Wuhan. *Journal of Allergy and Clinical Immunology,* 146(1), 110-118.

[217] Tang N, Li D, Wang X, Sun Z. "Abnormal coagulation parameters are associated with poor prognosis in patients with novel coronavirus pneumonia." *J Thromb Haemost.* 2020;18((4)):844–7.

[218] Berger, JS, Kunichoff, D, Adhikari, S, Ahuja, T, Amoroso, N, Aphinyanaphongs, Y, Horwitz, LI. (2020). Prevalence and outcomes of D-dimer elevation in hospitalized patients with COVID-19. *Arteriosclerosis, thrombosis, and vascular biology,* 40(10), 2539-2547.

[219] Siegal, DM, Barnes, GD, Langlois, NJ, Lee, A, Middeldorp, S, Skeith, L, Le Gal, G. (2020). A toolkit for the collection of thrombosis-related data elements in COVID-19 clinical studies. *Blood Advances,* 4(24), 6259-6273.

[220] Al-Samkari, H, Karp Leaf, RS, Dzik, WH, Carlson, JC, Fogerty, AE, Waheed, A, Rosovsky, RP. (2020). COVID-19 and coagulation: bleeding and thrombotic manifestations of SARS-CoV-2 infection. *Blood,* 136(4), 489-500.

[221] Iba, T, Levy, JH, Levi, M, Connors, JM, Thachil, J. (2020). Coagulopathy of coronavirus disease 2019. *Critical care medicine.*

[222] Helms, J, Tacquard, C, Severac, F, Leonard-Lorant, I, Ohana, M., Delabranche, X, Meziani, F. (2020). High risk of thrombosis in patients with severe SARS-CoV-2 infection: a multicenter prospective cohort study. *Intensive care medicine,* 46(6), 1089-1098.

[223] Zhang, L, Yan, X, Fan, Q, Liu, H, Liu, X, Liu, Z, Zhang, Z. (2020). D-dimer levels on admission to predict in-hospital mortality in patients with Covid-19. *Journal of thrombosis and haemostasis,* 18(6), 1324-1329.

[224] Ranucci, M, Ballotta, A, Di Dedda, U, Baryshnikova, E, Dei Poli, M, Resta, M, Menicanti, L. (2020). The procoagulant pattern of patients with COVID-19 acute respiratory distress syndrome. *Journal of Thrombosis and Haemostasis,* 18(7), 1747-1751.

[225] Canzano, P, Brambilla, M, Porro, B, Cosentino, N, Tortorici, E, Vicini, S, Camera, M. (2021). Platelet and endothelial activation as potential mechanisms behind the thrombotic complications of COVID-19 patients. *Basic to Translational Science,* 6(3), 202-218.

[226] Wada, H, Thachil, J, Di Nisio, M, Mathew, P, Kurosawa, S, Gando, S, Toh, CH. (2013). Guidance for diagnosis and treatment of disseminated intravascular coagulation from harmonization of the recommendations from three guidelines. *Journal of thrombosis and haemostasis,* 11(4), 761-767.

[227] Alhazzani, W, Møller, MH, Arabi, Y.M, Loeb, M, Gong, MN, Fan, E, Rhodes, A. (2020). Surviving Sepsis Campaign: guidelines on the management of critically ill adults with Coronavirus Disease 2019 (COVID-19*). Intensive care medicine,* 46(5), 854-887.

[228] Wiersinga, WJ., Rhodes, A, Cheng, AC, Peacock, SJ, Prescott, HC. (2020). Pathophysiology, transmission, diagnosis, and treatment of coronavirus disease 2019 (COVID-19): a review. *JAMA,* 324(8), 782-793.

[229] Mammen MJ, Aryal K, Alhazzani W, Alexander PE. "Corticosteroids for patients with acute respiratory distress syndrome: a systematic review and meta-analysis of randomized trials." *Polish Archives of Internal Medicine* 2020;130(4): 276-286.

[230] Karakike, E, Giamarellos-Bourboulis, EJ, Kyprianou, M., Fleischmann-Struzek, C, Pletz, MW, Netea, MG, Kyriazopoulou, E. (2021). Coronavirus disease 2019 as cause of viral sepsis: a systematic review and meta-analysis. *Critical care medicine,* 49(12), 2042.

[231] Campello, E, Bulato, C, Spiezia, L, Boscolo, A, Poletto, F, Cola, M, Simioni, P. (2021). Thrombin generation in patients with COVID-19 with and without thromboprophylaxis. *Clinical Chemistry and Laboratory Medicine (CCLM),* 59(7), 1323-1330.

[232] De La Morena-Barrio, ME, Bravo-Pérez, C, Miñano, A, De La Morena-Barrio, B, Fernandez-Perez, MP, Bernal, E, Lozano, ML. (2021). Prognostic value of thrombin generation parameters in hospitalized COVID-19 patients. *Scientific Reports,* 11(1), 1-11.

[233] Tang, N, Bai, H, Chen, X, Gong, J, Li, D, Sun, Z. (2020). Anticoagulant treatment is associated with decreased mortality in severe coronavirus disease 2019 patients with coagulopathy. *Journal of thrombosis and haemostasis,* 18(5), 1094-1099.

[234] Vaughn, VM, Yost, M, Abshire, C, Flanders, SA, Paje, D, Grant, P, Barnes, GD. (2021). Trends in venous thromboembolism anticoagulation in patients hospitalized with COVID-19. *JAMA network open,* 4(6), e2111788-e2111788.

[235] Paranjpe, I, Fuster, V, Lala, A, Russak, AJ, Glicksberg, BS, Levin, MA, Nadkarni, GN. (2020). Association of treatment dose anticoagulation with in-hospital survival among hospitalized patients with COVID-19. *Journal of the American College of Cardiology,* 76(1), 122-124.

[236] Gozzo, L, Viale, P, Longo, L, Vitale, DC, Drago, F. (2020). The potential role of heparin in patients with COVID-19: beyond the anticoagulant effect. *A review. Frontiers in pharmacology,* 11, 1307.

[237] Donato, AA. (2021). In non–critically ill patients with COVID-19, therapeutic anticoagulation improved survival to discharge without organ support. *Annals of Internal Medicine,* 174(12), JC134.

[238] Ten Cate, H. (2021). Surviving Covid-19 with heparin?. *New England Journal of Medicine,* 385(9), 845-846.

[239] Cuker, A, Tseng, EK, Nieuwlaat, R, Angchaisuksiri, P, Blair, C, Dane, K, Schünemann, HJ. (2022). American Society of Hematology living guidelines on the use of anticoagulation for thromboprophylaxis in patients with COVID-19: January 2022 update on the use of therapeutic-intensity anticoagulation in acutely ill patients. *Blood Advances,* 6(17), 4915-4923.

[240] Cui, S, Chen, S, Li, X, Liu, S, Wang, F. (2020). Prevalence of venous thromboembolism in patients with severe novel coronavirus pneumonia. *Journal of Thrombosis and Haemostasis,* 18(6), 1421-1424.

[241] Chow, JH, Khanna, AK, Kethireddy, S, Yamane, D, Levine, A, Jackson, AM, Mazzeffi, MA. (2021). Aspirin use is associated with decreased mechanical ventilation, intensive care unit admission, and in-hospital mortality in hospitalized patients with coronavirus disease 2019. *Anesthesia & Analgesia,* 132(4), 930-941.

[242] Mohamed-Hussein, AA, Aly, KM, Ibrahim, MEA. (2020). Should aspirin be used for prophylaxis of COVID-19-induced coagulopathy? *Medical Hypotheses,* 144, 109975.

[243] Wenzel, P, Daiber, A, Oelze, M, Brandt, M, Closs, E, Xu, J, Münzel, T. (2008). Mechanisms underlying recoupling of eNOS by HMG-CoA reductase inhibition in a rat model of streptozotocin-induced diabetes mellitus. *Atherosclerosis,* 198(1), 65-76.

[244] Kwak BR, Mulhaupt F, Mach F. "Atherosclerosis: anti-inflammatory and immunomodulatory activities of statins." *Autoimmun. Rev.* 2003;2(6):332–338.

[245] Zhang, XJ, Qin, JJ, Cheng, XU, Shen, L, Zhao, YC, Yuan, Y, Li, H. (2020). In-hospital use of statins is associated with a reduced risk of mortality among individuals with COVID-19. *Cell metabolism,* 32(2), 176-187.

[246] Güner, HR, Hasanoğlu, İ, Kayaaslan, B, Aypak, A, Kalem, AK, Eser, F, Dinc, B. (2020). COVID-19 experience of the major pandemic response center in the capital: results ofthe pandemic's first month in Turkey. *Turkish journal of medical sciences,* 50(8), 1801-1809.

[247] Tufan A, Avanoğlu Güler A, Matucci-Cerinic M. "COVID-19, immune system response, hyperinflammation and repurposing antirheumatic drugs." *Turkish Journal of Medical Science* 2020; 50(SI-1): 620-632.

[248] Cavalli, G, De Luca, G, Campochiaro, C, Della-Torre, E, Ripa, M, Canetti, D, Dagna, L. (2020). Interleukin-1 blockade with high-dose anakinra in patients with COVID-19, acute respiratory distress syndrome, and hyperinflammation: a retrospective cohort study. *The Lancet Rheumatology,* 2(6), e325-e331.

[249] Huet, T, Beaussier, H, Voisin, O, Jouveshomme, S, Dauriat, G., Lazareth, I., Hayem, G. (2020). Anakinra for severe forms of COVID-19: a cohort study. *The Lancet Rheumatology,* 2(7), e393-e400.

[250] Bronte, V, Ugel, S, Tinazzi, E, Vella, A, De Sanctis, F, Canè, S, Olivieri, O. (2020). Baricitinib restrains the immune dysregulation in patients with severe COVID-19. *The Journal of clinical investigatio*n, 130(12), 6409-6416.

Chapter 6

Vascularization and Cardiovascular Diseases

Esra Kansu Dinc*, MD
Dr. Halil İbrahim Özsoy Bolvadin State Hospital, Department of Cardiology, Afyonkarahisar, Turkey

Abstract

To understand the normal functions of vascular cells and how they are affected by various vascular movements, researchers and clinicians need to treat patients with peripheral artery disease, coronary artery disease, and hypertension. It is, therefore, essential to know the basic concepts of vascular diseases and to learn how common diseases change the foundations of vascular control. This chapter will provide an overview of the basic concepts of cardiovascular diseases.

Keywords: endothelial dysfunction, tissue engineering, endothelial cells, atherosclerosis, smooth muscle cells

Introduction

Most vessel wall cells comprise endothelial cells (EC) and smooth muscle cells (SMC). The rest of the wall contains an extracellular matrix containing elastin, collagen, and glycosaminoglycans. ECS and SMCs, the main cellular elements of the vascular wall, play a central role in vascular biology and pathology. These cells' integrated functions are essential in adapting the vascular bed to hemodynamic and biochemical stimuli.

---

* Corresponding Author's Email: dr.ekansu@hotmail.com.

In: Vascularization and Its Role in Medicine and Tissue Engineering
Editors: Emre Bulbul and Murat Oguz Ozilhan
ISBN: 979-8-89113-041-8

Normal EC function is crucial for vascular cell hemostasis. It is well known that diseases such as atherosclerosis result from endothelial dysfunction. Usually, the endothelium has three main parts: 1) it is metabolically active secretory tissue. 2) acts as an anticoagulant, antithrombotic surface. 3) it acts as a barrier preventing the indiscriminate passage of blood components into the arterial wall. Endothelial damage plays a role in many pathologies such as thrombosis, atherosclerosis, and hypertensive vascular lesions [1].

SMCs, the second major cell type in the standard arterial wall, have many essential roles in normal vascular homeostasis, as a therapeutic target in cardiovascular medicine, and in the pathogenesis of arterial disease. These cells contract and relax, controlling blood flow in various vascular beds. However, in larger arteries involved in atherosclerosis, smooth muscle contraction may lead to vasospasm as a complication of atherosclerosis that will result in decreased blood flow. Smooth muscle cells are crucial in forming atherosclerotic lesions and their complications. These cells can migrate and proliferate, causing the formation of intimal hyperplastic lesions, including atherosclerosis and restenosis or anastomotic hyperplasia, as a complication of vein grafts. The death of smooth muscle cells triggers the destabilization of atheromatous plaques, leading to ectatic remodeling and, ultimately, aneurysm formation [2].

Atherosclerosis

Atherosclerosis is a pathological process that can cause coronary, cerebral, peripheral artery, and aortic diseases [3]. Atherosclerosis is an inflammatory and fibroproliferative response to plasma-derived atherogenic lipoprotein deposition in the arterial intima [4].

Arteries morphologically consist of the intima, media, and adventitia layers. The intima layer forms the luminal surface of the arterial wall. A single line of endothelial cells continuously covering the luminal surface is the essential part of the intima layer.

Atherosclerosis is an intimal disease of large and medium-sized arteries such as the aorta, coronary, iliofemoral, carotid (bifurcation), and, to a lesser extent, intracranial arteries. Although the reason is not fully understood, scientific studies have proven that some arterial structures (such as the internal mammary artery) resist this condition. Intramyocardial arteries are similarly resistant to atherosclerosis. On the other hand, epicardial coronary arteries are the vascular structures in our body that are most prone to atherosclerosis [5].

Atherosclerosis, the pathological basis of coronary artery disease, usually begins in childhood. It is a progressive disease with clinical manifestations in middle and late adulthood [6]. According to the results obtained from autopsies, it was observed that atherosclerotic plaque formation followed a series of events [7]. The frequent presence of fatty streaks in the coronary arteries in children suggests that they are the first step in developing atherosclerotic plaque. The most common sites of fatty streaks in the twenties are the proximal segment of the left anterior descending coronary artery (LAD). All types of plaque can be seen in many people of advancing age. This process continues throughout life [7, 8].

Histopathology

Fatty streaks seen in the earliest stage of atherosclerosis are focal thickenings due to the increase in smooth muscle cells and extracellular matrix in the intima layer. Foam cells formed after oxidative modification of low-density lipoprotein (LDL) and endocytosis by monocyte-derived macrophages cause fatty streaks. Studies have shown that fatty streaks begin to include in the aorta at the end of the first decade of life, the coronary arteries in the second decade, and the intima layers of the cerebral arteries in the third decade. Since these lines are not stenotic, they are asymptomatic.

Migration of fibroblasts and smooth muscle cells into fatty streaks occurs due to disruption of endothelial integrity and cytokines released from inflammatory cells. As a result of the proliferation of these cells, fibrous plaques are formed [8]. Fibrous plaques cause symptomatically significant arterial lumen narrowing but do not lead to significant clinical events unless they rupture [9].

Complicated lesions consist of a lipid core that accounts for more than 40% of the plaque volume. Calcification, neovascularization, ulceration, erosion, and rupture can be seen in these plaques [10]. Microvessels cause intraplaque bleeding, and therefore, inflammatory cell migration is accelerated. As a result, dynamic and complex events follow each other in atherosclerosis [11].

Lipid core size and fibrous cap thickness are significant determinants of plaque stability. Plaque stability is directly proportional to the fibrous cap. As the fibrous cap thickens, plaque stability increases; however, as the lipid content increases, the plaque becomes unstable [9]. Compared to stable plaques, increased matrix metalloproteinase activation, neovascularization, and positive remodeling are observed in sensitive plaques. These plaques are more likely to rupture and cause the acute coronary syndrome. Coronary atherosclerosis-related morbidity and mortality are mainly due to these complicated lesions [10].

Etiopathogenesis

Many factors contribute to the pathogenesis of atherosclerosis, including endothelial dysfunction, inflammatory and immunological factors, dyslipidemia, plaque rupture, and smoking.

The endothelium forms a functional biological interface between blood and all other tissues. It regulates tone, growth, hemostasis, and inflammation throughout the vessel. Vasodilator dysfunction in the endothelium is the first step in atherosclerosis and is thought to be mainly due to endothelial-derived nitric oxide loss [12].

Endothelial dysfunction is associated with many risk factors that cause atherosclerosis, including hypercholesterolemia, diabetes, hypertension, and smoking. Endothelial dysfunction is specifically induced by oxidized LDL, and this can be considered a final common pathway [13]. With endothelial dysfunction, monocytes attach to the endothelium, triggering inflammation and forming atherosclerotic plaque. Endothelial dysfunction is the first step in the attachment and progression of lesions in the atherosclerosis process [14].

Evidence of inflammation in atherosclerotic lesions has been noted in histological observations, and inflammation is critical for recognizing the pathogenesis of atherosclerosis [15, 16]. After taking up oxidized LDL, macrophages release various inflammatory mediators, cytokines, and growth factors [17]. Molecules involved in inflammation are known as monocyte chemotactic protein (MCP)-1, intercellular adhesion molecule (ICAM)-1, macrophage and granulocyte-macrophage colony-stimulating factors, CD40 ligand, interleukin (IL)-1, IL-3, IL-6, IL-8 and tumor necrosis factor (TNF) alpha [18, 19]. High-sensitivity C-reactive protein (hs-CRP) is one of the indicators of inflammation. Although genetic data do not support hs-CRP function as a causal risk factor, it does help that it is associated with an increased risk of atherosclerotic cardiovascular disease, independent of cholesterol level [20]. Hs-CRP has been recognized as a valuable marker for identifying individuals with increased vascular inflammation [21].

Dyslipidemia plays an essential role in the development of atherosclerosis. Experiments in animals have shown accelerated atherosclerosis with a high-cholesterol diet. Epidemiological studies have shown an increased incidence of atherosclerosis when serum cholesterol concentrations are above 150 mg/dL (3.9 mmol/L) [22]. High LDL cholesterol (LDL-C) level is a significant risk factor for atherosclerosis [23].

Cholesterol accumulates in lipid-laden macrophages (foam cells) and lipid cores within atherosclerotic plaque [24]. Accumulation of LDL-C in foam cells leads to mitochondrial dysfunction, apoptosis, and necrosis. As a result, cellular proteases, inflammatory cytokines, and prothrombotic molecules are released [25]. Much of the evidence accumulated over the past 50 years has shown that lowering LDL-C can reduce cardiovascular events and lower LDL-C levels are associated with a better clinical outcome [26].

Unlike LDL-C, high-density lipoprotein (HDL) cholesterol has antiatherogenic properties such as preservation of endothelial function and anti-thrombogenic effect. There is an inverse relationship between plasma HDL cholesterol levels and cardiovascular risk. Low (<40 mg/dl) HDL cholesterol levels are a risk factor for coronary artery disease (CAD). High (>60 mg/dl) HDL cholesterol levels are a protective factor for CAD [27].

Observational and genetic studies have revealed a causal relationship between atherosclerotic cardiovascular diseases and lipoprotein (Lp)(a). While the LDL part of Lp(a) increases atherosclerosis, the plasminogen-like apo(a) molecule inhibits fibrinolysis and causes thrombus accumulation [28]. Lp(a) initiates signaling pathways in vascular endothelial cells, leading to proatherogenic changes. Lp(a) is associated with an increased risk of cardiovascular events in some studies [29].

Hypertension is a significant risk factor for the development of atherosclerosis, mainly coronary and cerebral circulation [30]. Elevated blood pressure causes changes in the surface of the intima layer and increases lipid infiltration, thus leading to the microthrombus formation and accelerating atherogenesis [31]. Many studies have proven that high blood pressure is a risk factor for atherosclerotic cardiovascular diseases [27].

Smoking is another crucial risk factor for atherosclerosis. It is highly thrombogenic and affects all stages of atherosclerosis, from endothelial dysfunction to acute clinical events. Cigarette smoke exposure inhibits endothelium-dependent vasodilation through nitric oxide (NO) reduction. Cigarette smoking is associated with increased levels of multiple inflammatory markers, including C-reactive protein (CRP), IL-6, and TNF alpha, in both male and female smokers [32]. Smoking increases fibrinogen levels, decreases fibrinolysis, and increases oxidized LDL [33].

Diabetes mellitus (DM) is one of the most important risk factors for developing atherosclerotic cardiovascular diseases. It has been observed that endothelial dysfunction and accelerated atherosclerosis in patients followed up with DM play an essential role in developing macrovascular complications. In diabetic patients, low HDL cholesterol levels are observed, while high triglyceride and atherogenic small and dense LDL cholesterol particles are observed [34]. Atherosclerosis and type 2 DM share common pathological mechanisms, including elevation of the inflammatory cytokines MCP-1 and IL-6 [35].

In addition to traditional risk factors, many other factors are thought to play a role in the etiopathogenesis of atherosclerosis. These are tissue factors, angiotensin-2, endothelin-1, various adhesion molecules, flow characteristics in arteries, mitochondrial deoxyribonucleic acid (DNA) damage, chronic infections (Chlamydia pneumonia, Cytomegalovirus, coxsackie B, Helicobacter pylori), and genetic predispositions [36-40].

Atherosclerosis is asymptomatic until plaque stenosis exceeds 70 or 80 per cent of the lumen diameter. This may produce a reduction in coronary blood flow to the myocardium. These stenotic lesions may produce typical angina pectoris symptoms. The progression of atherosclerotic plaques involves two different processes. These are a chronic process that causes slow vessel lumen narrowing and an acute process that causes rapid luminal occlusion associated with plaque bleeding and/or luminal thrombosis [41].

Atherosclerosis Complications

Arterial Stenoses

Narrowing of the arterial lumen begins when the burden of atherosclerotic plaque exceeds the outward remodeling capacity of the artery. In the chronic asymptomatic or stable phase of lesion development, growth probably continues with rapid progressions followed by relatively quiet periods. Eventually, the stenoses reach a size that impairs blood flow from the artery. Lesions that produce more than 60% stenosis restrict blood flow in case of increased demand. This type of atherosclerotic disease often makes chronic stable angina pectoris or intermittent claudication with increased need [2].

Thrombosis and Complication of Atheroma

In developing acute coronary syndromes, thrombosis is the critical mechanism in transitioning from chronic to acute atherosclerosis. Understanding of the mechanisms of coronary thrombosis has advanced markedly. We now know that the physical rupture of atherosclerotic plaque often leads to acute thrombosis [42]. The primary mechanism responsible for two-thirds of acute myocardial infarctions is the rupture of the fibrous capsule. Superficial erosion of the intima is another mechanism responsible for a quarter of acute myocardial infarctions in selected reference cases of sudden cardiac death. Superficial erosion is a more common mechanism of sudden coronary death in women than in men [43].

Plaque Rupture and Thrombosis

The rupture of the fibrous cap of the plaque reflects an imbalance between the forces that stretch the plaque capsule and the strength of the fibrous capsule. Interstitial forms of collagen constitute most of the biomechanical resistance to fibrous capsular rupture. Therefore, collagen metabolism probably regulates the susceptibility of the plaque to rupture.

Factors that reduce collagen synthesis by SMCs may also impair the repair and maintenance of the fibrous capsule of the plaque. In addition, increased catabolism of the extracellular matrix macromolecules that make up the fibrous capsule may contribute to the weakening of this structure and its susceptibility to rupture and thrombosis. Thinning of the fibrous capsule of the plaque due to decreased collagen synthesis and increased degradation explains that histological studies show a thin fibrous capsule in atherosclerotic plaques that have likely ruptured and resulted in a fatal myocardial infarction [44].

Another feature of sensitive plaque, identified by the pathological analysis, is the relative absence of SMCs. Since these cells synthesize new collagen necessary for the repair and maintenance of the fibrous capsule matrix, their lack may contribute to the weakening of the fibrous capsule and, therefore, susceptibility to plaque rupture [45].

Significant macrophage accumulation and a large pool of lipids are the third microanatomical feature of fragile atherosclerotic plaque. The success of lipid-lowering therapy in reducing the incidence of acute myocardial infarction and unstable angina may be due to reduced lipid accumulation and inflammation, and reduction in plaque thrombogenicity [46].

Thrombosis Due to Superficial Erosion of Plaque

In humans, superficial erosion is more likely to cause fatal acute myocardial infarction in women, hypertriglyceridemia, and diabetic persons, but the underlying cause is unknown.

Most plaque ruptures do not result in clinically significant coronary events. Careful pathoanatomical examinations of hearts from people who died due to non-cardiac death showed a surprisingly high incidence of plaque rupture and limited mural thrombi. In patients with severe but chronic stable coronary atherosclerosis undergoing heart transplantation for ischemic cardiomyopathy, sustained but asymptomatic plaque ruptures have been observed in immediately re-fixed hearts [2].

Inflammation in Atherogenesis

Studies in the autopsy of atherosclerotic plaques that cause fatal thrombosis have highlighted sensitive high-risk plaque. Studies in the autopsy of atherosclerotic plaques that cause fatal thrombosis have highlighted sensitive high-risk plaque. This observation has prompted the search for many ways to detect and treat such highly atherosclerotic lesions. Current evidence indicates that such high-risk plaques are found in more than one place in a coronary tree [47, 48]. Inflammation, characteristic of these plaques described as sensitive, seems widespread. Careful examination of angiographies of individuals with the acute coronary syndrome has shown evidence of plaque ulceration and thrombosis at multiple sites in these cases. Individuals with more than one unstable lesion, according to angiographic criteria, tend to have a worse outcome during follow-up. Intravascular ultrasound, optical coherence tomography, magnetic resonance imaging, and computed tomography have provided a better understanding of the morphology of plaques that cause acute coronary syndromes [49].

Much concordant evidence supports inflammation's systemic and diffuse nature in patients with acute coronary syndrome [50]. Several studies have shown that various markers of systemic inflammation, such as C-reactive protein, are elevated in individuals at risk for acute coronary syndrome. Experiments using imaging studies and inflammatory markers support the nature of diffuse and systemic instability of atheromas in individuals with or at risk of acute coronary syndrome. Recognition of this condition has important implications for treatment. These patients should receive systemic therapy to stabilize multiple high-risk lesions that may lead to recurrent events, in addition to appropriately used local revascularization therapies [2].

Special Conditions of Arteriosclerosis

Restenosis

Restenosis is a healing response that includes complex molecular and cellular events that develop in the damaged artery wall after percutaneous coronary intervention (PCI) [Figure 1 and Figure 2]. Coronary stent restenosis is defined in three different ways [51].

- Histological Restenosis: Restenosis occurs at the cellular level in the vascular lumen and can be detected by intravascular ultrasonography (IVUS).
- Clinical Restenosis: Revascularization of the target artery or lesion or recurrence of symptoms and signs of ischemia (at rest or with stress) requiring medical treatment.
- Angiographic Restenosis: It was determined as 50% or more stenosis within the stent or up to 5 mm outside the proximal or distal segment from the edges of the stent. It is defined by the presence of one of three criteria:
    1) Re-stenosis of 50% or more in the arterial lumen compared to the standard lumen diameter in the adjacent vessel segment after PCI to the coronary artery,
    2) Loss of more than 50% of the lumen gained,
    3) It is defined as stenosis that decreases below 50% after PCI and 70% or more stenosis in the control [51, 52].

Pseudorestenosis is the name given to a certain amount of narrowing in the arterial lumen due to elastic recoil in the first minutes due to insufficient dilatation in 15% of dilated stenoses during PCI. In this case, the probability of developing real restenosis after six months is also higher [53].

The reduction in lumen diameter after stent implantation occurs due to neointimal tissue proliferation secondary to damage to the arterial tissue during PCI [54]. Many thrombogenic, mitogenic, and vasoactive substances are released during this process. Many factors, primarily arterial remodeling, and neointimal hyperplasia, play a role in the pathophysiology [55].

Arterial remodeling: At the onset of atherosclerosis, the plaque pushes the external elastic membrane outward without narrowing the vessel's cross-sectional area with positive vascular remodeling. On the other hand, in the restenotic process, adverse remodeling is observed. Collagen replaces hyaluronic acid in the extracellular matrix. As a result, adverse vessel wall remodelling develops with adventitia layer thickening and wound contraction [51].

Neointimal hyperplasia: During PCI, platelet adhesion, activation, and plaque rupture due to barotrauma are stimulated. Mitogens such as thromboxane A2, serotonin, and platelet-derived growth factor (PDGF) are released from platelets. As a result of these secreted mitogens, the proliferation of SMCs and migration to the intima are stimulated. Levels of mitogenic proto-oncogenes increase in SMCs, and thus the cells function as synthesis rather than contraction [56]. As a result, the activated SMCs proliferate and migrate to the intima layer. They cause neointima development with the increase of extracellular matrix and collagen. Myofibroblasts in the adventitia can also migrate to the intima. Nitrous oxide released from intact endothelium inhibits SMC growth, while endothelial dysfunction contributes to SMC proliferation and migration [55].

Neointimal hyperplasia is the leading cause of stent restenosis and is composed of smooth muscle cells and an extracellular matrix. Neointima development is observed at a high level until the sixth month. Between six months and three years, it slows down. Examples of intra-stent restenosis lesions are hypocellular compared to angioplasty restenosis. In addition, compared to primary plaques, the cell coverage is less, and the collagen and proteoglycan matrix content is higher [51].

Elastic shrinkage (Recoil): The coronary arteries' elastic membranes contain many elastic fibers. As the balloon is inflated, these fibers are stretched and contract rapidly upon deflating. They cause about 40% loss in the lumen. It mainly affects the restenosis mechanism that develops after balloon angioplasty. Stents significantly reduce this phenomenon.

Thrombus organization: As a result of PCI, disruption of the endothelium and dissection of the media layer occurs. Platelet adhesion and aggregation occur due to the release of subintimal substances such as collagen, fibronectin, laminin, and the von Willebrand factor. Fibrin and platelets accumulate on the stent struts. The association of platelets and fibrins in the stent restenosis area with neovascularization and neointimal thickening indicates that the formation of a mural thrombus may contribute to restenosis [55]. It is known that thrombus development is more prominent in patients with other diseases, such as DM.

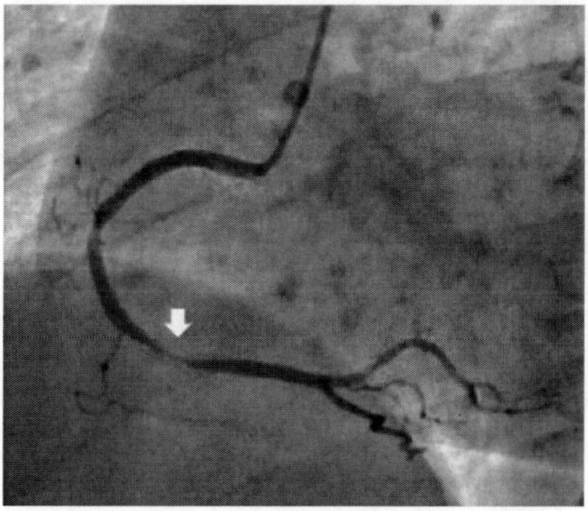

Figure 1. Diffuse type in-stent restenosis in the right coronary artery.

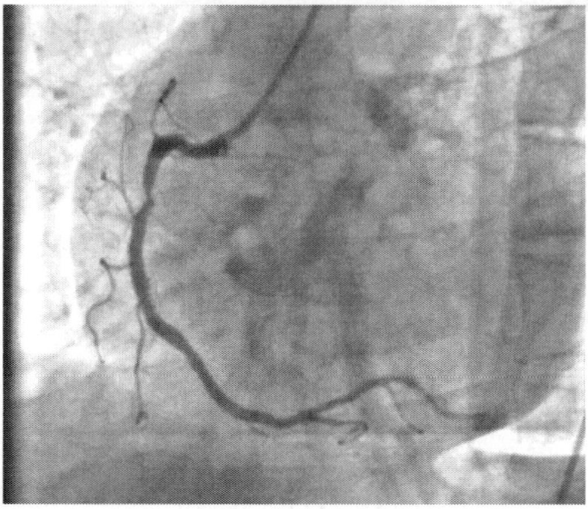

Figure 2. Focal type in-stent restenosis in the right coronary artery.

Resolution of inflammation: During stent implantation, a close relationship has been shown between stent restenosis and penetration of lipid content and inflammation in case of media layer injury. Since inflammatory cells, especially macrophages, play a role in all stages of stent restenosis, the resolution of inflammation is essential in restenosis [51].

Accelerated Atherosclerosis after Transplantation

After the development of effective immunosuppressive therapies such as cyclosporine, the main limitation to the long-term survival of cardiac allografts is due to accelerated arterial hyperplastic disease. The term arteriosclerosis rather than atherosclerosis is preferred to describe this process because the description of this process is unrelated to lipids. This type of arterial disease often presents a diagnostic challenge. The patient may not show typical anginal symptoms due to post-transplant cardiac denervation. In addition, graft coronary disease is concentric and diffuse, affecting the proximal epicardial coronary vessels and small intramyocardial branches. Therefore, angiography, highly suitable for imaging focal and eccentric stenoses, underestimates the extent of transplantation arteriosclerosis.

The majority of patients undergoing transplantation have atherosclerotic disease and ischemic cardiomyopathy. However, a substantial minority undergoes heart transplants for dilated cardiomyopathy, and almost all patients have no atherosclerotic risk factors. Despite traditional risk factors, this group shares the same risk for developing accelerated arteriosclerosis. This observation suggests that this type of accelerated arteriosclerosis's pathophysiology differs from typical atherosclerosis.

Significant data from both human and experimental studies suggest that immunological differences between host and recipient vessels may play a role in the pathogenesis of the disease [57].

Aneurysmal Disease

Atherosclerosis can also cause aneurysmal disease. In particular, aneurysmal disease characteristically affects the infrarenal abdominal aorta. This area is highly prone to the development of atherosclerosis. The relative blood scarcity of the tunica media in this part of the abdominal aorta due to the absence of the vasa vasorum may explain the regional predisposition to aneurysm formation in this part of the arterial tree. In addition, a bipedal human's lumbar lordosis can alter the distal aorta's hydrodynamics and produce flow disturbances that lead to lesion formation.

In typical coronary atherosclerosis, the enlargement of the intimal lesion creates the stenotic lesion. The tunica media underlying the enlarged intima is generally thinned, but the overall structure remains well preserved. Conversely, transmural disruption of arterial architecture is observed in aneurysmal disease. In particular, the laminar structure of the well-circumscribed regular tunica media is lost with the destruction of the elastic lamina. Medial SMCs, well preserved in typical stenotic lesions, draw attention with their rarity in the media of advanced aortic aneurysms.

While studies of the pathophysiology underlying these anatomical-pathological findings are disappointing, most studies have shown that matrix-destroying proteinases, including matrix metalloproteinases, are overexpressed in human aortic aneurysm preparations [58]. Thus, increased elastolysis may explain the disruption of the tunica media structure, which is usually regular in this disease. In addition, aortic aneurysms show significant evidence of inflammation, particularly in the adventitia. It is thought that inflammatory mediators such as lymphocytes, soluble cytokines, and Fas ligand, which are characteristically abundant in the adventitial side of the aneurysmal region, may contribute to SMC apoptosis, SMC destruction, and aneurysm formation. Although extracellular matrix destruction and SMC death occur where atherosclerosis leads to stenosis, for unknown reasons, they occur especially at sites of aneurysm formation and affect the tunica media more widely [2].

Hypertension

Hypertension is characterized by dysfunction of vascular smooth muscle and endothelium. In chronic hypertension, endothelium-dependent relaxations are inhibited, and endothelium-derived contractile activity is increased [59, 60]. Hypertension also causes an increase in vessel wall mass. Vascular remodeling involves two stages. Reversible intense vasoconstriction mediated by an initial neural or endogenous signal is followed by vessel wall remodeling characterized by increased smooth muscle mass gain and vessel lumen narrowing. Thus, increased vascular tone and remodeling of vessels lead to an increase in systemic vascular resistance that increases hypertensive syndromes [1].

Cardiovascular Tissue Engineering

Tissue engineering aims to produce new tissue scaffolds specific to the geometry of damaged or dysfunctional tissue/organ structures and to create artificial tissue compatible with the body. It can fulfill the function of the tissue/organ. Cardiovascular diseases are among the leading causes of death in adults with high mortality. Treatment of cardiovascular diseases is limited due to factors such as donor deficiency and immune tolerance. Therefore, studies on personalized treatment methods are continuing rapidly. With the developments in biomaterials science and applications made with existing cell studies, tissue engineering studies are gaining momentum daily. Cardiovascular tissue engineering has been one of the priority targets in tissue engineering studies from the beginning in terms of application and treatment [61].

Clinically appropriately sized designed tissues require a network of vessels to supply cells with nutrients and oxygen. Including a vascular network before implantation can assist this need by connecting to the patient's vasculature.

A highly organized vasculature is required to provide adequate nutrition to all cells and to connect successfully to the patient's vasculature. The initial organization of vascular networks can be designed and controlled using microfabrication technology such as photopatterning and bioprinting.

The geometry of vascular networks can also be controlled by adapting local microenvironments. Mechanical signals, fluid flows, or growth factors lead to the directed vascular organization.

A network connecting to the patient's vasculature after implantation can be incorporated during in vitro culture. This network needs to be highly organized for optimal integration, including venules, capillaries, and arterioles, to provide adequate nutrition to all cells. Because of the importance of vascularization for the clinical applicability of tissue engineering, many approaches have been explored to incorporate an organized vascular network into tissue structures [62].

Cardiovascular tissue studies aim to create structures with growth capacity, non-immunogenic and functionally supporting tissue and organ function. Its advantages over currently used prostheses are the improvements in tissue-engineered heart valves, vessels, and myocardial patches for repairing congenital heart anomalies, and the treatment of heart valve diseases or ischemic heart disease [63].

Conclusion

Identifying the molecular and cellular basis for dysfunction of the arterial wall in molecular diseases leads to developing clinical strategies for treating the patient and providing critical insights for new treatment targets. It is known that various risk factors for vascular diseases compromise both endothelial and smooth muscle function. More research is needed to determine at a more fundamental level the molecular events that link these risk factors to these diseases. Therapeutic approaches will become increasingly molecularly targeted. In addition, with the advent of stem cell technology, new doors will be opened for treatment. Once researchers understand the control mechanisms of stem cell targeting and differentiation, genetic and pharmacological manipulation of these cells could be the treatment of the future.

Cardiovascular applications with a tissue engineering approach in tissue damage treatments lead the way regarding clinical applications. Designing the optimal and functional vascular network will be essential for repairing congenital heart anomalies and treating heart valve diseases or ischemic heart disease.

References

[1] Basta, G. (2021). Direct or indirect endothelial damage? An unresolved question. *EBioMedicine*, 64.

[2] Burris, A. C., Shoukfeh, M. (2015). Basic coronary artery anatomy and histology. *Interventional Cardiology Imaging: An Essential Guide,* 1-12.

[3] Faxon, D. P., Fuster, V., Libby, P., Beckman, J. A., Hiatt, W. R., Thompson, R. W., Loscalzo, J. (2004). Atherosclerotic vascular disease conference: writing group III: pathophysiology. *Circulation*, 109(21), 2617-2625.

[4] Davies M J. Coronary artery remodelling and the assessment of stenosis by pathologists. *Histopathology*. 1998 Dec;33(6):497–500.

[5] Berliner, J. A., Navab, M., Fogelman, A. M., Frank, J. S., Demer, L. L., Edwards, P. A., Lusis, A. J. (1995). Atherosclerosis: basic mechanisms: oxidation, inflammation, and genetics. *Circulation*, 91(9), 2488-2496.

[6] Lorkowski S, Cullen P. Atherosclerosis: Pathogenesis, Clinical Features and Treatment. *Encycl. Life Sci.* 2007;1–11.

[7] Stary H C. Evolution and progression of atherosclerotic lesions in coronary arteries of children and young adults. *Arteriosclerosis.* 1989;9(1 Suppl):I19-32.

[8] Ross R. The pathogenesis of atherosclerosis: a perspective for the 1990s. *Nature.* 1993 Apr;362(6423):801–9.

[9] Zengin, H. (2012). Ateroskleroz patogenezi (Pathogenesis of atherosclerosis) *Journal of experimental and clinical medicine*, 29(3s), 101-106.

[10] Shanahan C M, Cary N R B, Metcalfe J C, Weissberg PL. High expression of genes for calcification-regulating proteins in human atherosclerotic plaques. *J. Clin. Invest.* 1994;93(6):2393–402.

[11] Aikawa, M., Sugiyama, S., Hill, C. C., Voglic, S. J., Rabkin, E., Fukumoto, Y., Libby, P. (2002). Lipid lowering reduces oxidative stress and endothelial cell activation in rabbit atheroma. *Circulation,* 106(11), 1390-1396.

[12] Kitta, Y., Obata, J. E., Nakamura, T., Hirano, M., Kodama, Y., Fujioka, D., Kugiyama, K. (2009). Persistent impairment of endothelial vasomotor function has a negative impact on outcome in patients with coronary artery disease. *Journal of the American College of Cardiology,* 53(4), 323-330.

[13] Anderson, T. J., Meredith, I. T., Charbonneau, F., Yeung, A. C., Frei, B., Selwyn, A. P., Ganz, P. (1996). Endothelium-dependent coronary vasomotion relates to the susceptibility of LDL to oxidation in humans. *Circulation,* 93(9), 1647-1650.

[14] Cominacini, L., Pasini, A. F., Garbin, U., Davoli, A., Tosetti, M. L., Campagnola, M., Sawamura, T. (2000). Oxidized low density lipoprotein (ox-LDL) binding to ox-LDL receptor-1 in endothelial cells induces the activation of NF-κB through an increased production of intracellular reactive oxygen species. *Journal of Biological Chemistry*, 275(17), 12633-12638.

[15] Paoletti R, Gotto A M J, Hajjar D P. Inflammation in atherosclerosis and implications for therapy. *Circulation.* 2004 Jun;109(23 Suppl 1):III20-6.

[16] Weber C, Noels H. Atherosclerosis: current pathogenesis and therapeutic options. *Nat, Med.* 2011 Nov;17(11):1410–1422.

[17] Steinberg D, Witztum J L. Oxidized low-density lipoprotein and atherosclerosis. *Arterioscler. Thromb. Vasc. Biol.* 2010 Dec;30(12):2311–2316.

[18] Ridker P M, Hennekens C H, Buring J E, Rifai N. C-reactive protein and other markers of inflammation in the prediction of cardiovascular disease in women. *N. Engl. J. Med.* 2000 Mar;342(12):836–843.

[19] Kaartinen M, Penttila A, Kovanen PT. Mast cells in rupture-prone areas of human coronary atheromas produce and store TNF-alpha. *Circulation.* 1996 Dec;94 (11):2787–2792.

[20] Ridker P M, Cushman M, Stampfer M J, Tracy R P, Hennekens CH. Inflammation, aspirin, and the risk of cardiovascular disease in apparently healthy men. *N. Engl. J. Med.* 1997 Apr;336(14):973–979.

[21] Ridker, P. M., Danielson, E., Fonseca, F. A., Genest, J., Gotto Jr, A. M., Kastelein, J. J., Glynn, R. J. (2008). Rosuvastatin to prevent vascular events in men and women with elevated C-reactive protein. *New England journal of medicine,* 359(21), 2195-2207.

[22] Stamler J, Wentworth D, Neaton J D. Is relationship between serum cholesterol and risk of premature death from coronary heart disease continuous and graded? Findings in 356,222 primary screenees of the Multiple Risk Factor Intervention Trial (MRFIT). *JAMA.* 1986 Nov 28;256(20):2823–2828.

[23] Gordon T, Castelli W P, Hjortland M C, Kannel W B, Dawber T R. High density lipoprotein as a protective factor against coronary heart disease. The Framingham Study. *Am. J. Med.* 1977 May;62(5):707–714.

[24] Iuliano L, Mauriello A, Sbarigia E, Spagnoli LG, Violi F. Radiolabeled native low-density lipoprotein injected into patients with carotid stenosis accumulates in macrophages of atherosclerotic plaque: effect of vitamin E supplementation. *Circulation.* 2000 Mar 21;101(11):1249–1254.

[25] Tabas I. Consequences of cellular cholesterol accumulation: basic concepts and physiological implications. *J. Clin. Invest.* 2002 Oct;110(7):905–911.

[26] Silverman, M. G., Ference, B. A., Im, K., Wiviott, S. D., Giugliano, R. P., Grundy, S. M., Sabatine, M. S. (2016). Association between lowering LDL-C and cardiovascular risk reduction among different therapeutic interventions: a systematic review and meta-analysis. *Jama*, 316(12), 1289-1297.

[27] Goodman D S, Hulley S B, Clark L T, Davis C E, Fuster V, LaRosa J C, Oberman A, Schaefer E J, Steinberg D, Brown W V, Grundy S M. Report of the National Cholesterol Education Program Expert Panel on detection, evaluation, and treatment of high blood cholesterol in adults. *Archives of Internal Medicine.* 1988 Jan 1;148(1):36-69.

[28] Boffa M B, Koschinsky M L. Update on lipoprotein(a) as a cardiovascular risk factor and mediator. *Curr. Atheroscler. Rep.* 2013 Oct;15(10):360.

[29] Cho T, Romagnuolo R, Scipione C, Boffa MB, Koschinsky ML. Apolipoprotein(a) stimulates nuclear translocation of β-catenin: a novel pathogenic mechanism for lipoprotein(a). *Mol. Biol. Cell.* 2012/12/14. 2013 Feb;24(3):210–21.

[30] Frohlich J, Al-Sarraf A. Cardiovascular risk and atherosclerosis prevention. *Cardiovasc. Pathol.* 2012/04/12. 2013;22(1):16–8.

[31] Helgeland A, Hjermann I, Leren P, Enger S, Holme I. High-density lipoprotein cholesterol and antihypertensive drugs: the Oslo study. *Br. Med. J.* 1978 Aug 5;2(6134):403.

[32] Bermudez E A, Rifai N, Buring J E, Manson J E, Ridker P M. Relation between markers of systemic vascular inflammation and smoking in women. *Am. J. Cardiol.* 2002 May 1;89(9):1117–9.

[33] Nishio E, Watanabe Y. Cigarette smoke extract inhibits plasma paraoxonase activity by modification of the enzyme's free thiols. *Biochem. Biophys. Res. Commun.* 1997 Jul 18;236(2):289–93.

[34] Cavanaugh K L. Health literacy in diabetes care: explanation, evidence and equipment. *Diabetes management* (London, England). 2011 Mar;1(2):191.

[35] Park Y M, Kashyap S, Major J, Silverstein R L. Insulin promotes macrophage foam cell formation: potential implications in diabetes-related atherosclerosis. *Lab Invest.* 2012/04/23. 2012 Aug;92(8):1171–1180.

[36] Daugherty A, Manning MW, Cassis L A. Angiotensin II promotes atherosclerotic lesions and aneurysms in apolipoprotein E-deficient mice. *J. Clin. Invest.* 2000 Jun;105(11):1605–1612.

[37] Mathew V, Cannan C R, Miller V M, Barber D A, Hasdai D, Schwartz R S, Holmes Jr DR, Lerman A. Enhanced endothelin-mediated coronary vasoconstriction and attenuated basal nitric oxide activity in experimental hypercholesterolemia. *Circulation*. 1997 Sep 16;96(6):1930-1936.

[38] Yu E, Mercer J, Bennett M. Mitochondria in vascular disease. *Cardiovasc. Res.* 2012/03/05. 2012 Jul 15;95(2):173–182.

[39] Hagiwara H, Mitsumata M, Yamane T, Jin X, Yoshida Y. Laminar shear stress-induced GRO mRNA and protein expression in endothelial cells. *Circulation*. 1998 Dec 8;98(23):2584–2590.

[40] Patel P, Mendall M A, Carrington D, Strachan D P, Leatham E, Molineaux N, Levy J, Blakeston C, Seymour CA, Camm AJ, Northfield TC. Association of Helicobacter pylori and Chlamydia pneumoniae infections with coronary heart disease and cardiovascular risk factors. *BMJ*. 1995 Sep 16;311(7007):711-714.

[41] Falk E, Shah P K, Fuster V. Coronary plaque disruption. *Circulation*. 1995 Aug 1;92(3):657–671.

[42] Virmani R, Burke A P, Farb A, Kolodgie F D. Pathology of the vulnerable plaque. *J. Am. Coll. Cardiol.* 2006 Apr;47(8 Suppl):13-18.

[43] Kramer, M. C., Rittersma, S. Z., de Winter, R. J., Ladich, E. R., Fowler, D. R., Liang, Y. H., Virmani, R. (2010). Relationship of thrombus healing to underlying plaque morphology in sudden coronary death. *Journal of the American College of Cardiology*, 55(2), 122-132.

[44] Libby P. The molecular mechanisms of the thrombotic complications of atherosclerosis. *J. Intern. Med.* 2008 May;263(5):517–527.

[45] Clarke, M. C., Littlewood, T. D., Figg, N., Maguire, J. J., Davenport, A. P., Goddard, M., Bennett, M. R. (2008). Chronic apoptosis of vascular smooth muscle cells accelerates atherosclerosis and promotes calcification and medial degeneration. *Circulation research,* 102(12), 1529-1538.

[46] Libby P. Molecular and cellular mechanisms of the thrombotic complications of atherosclerosis. *J. Lipid. Res.* 2009 Apr;50 Suppl(Suppl):352-357.

[47] Libby P. Act local, act global: inflammation and the multiplicity of "vulnerable" coronary plaques. Vol. 45, *Journal of the American College of Cardiology*. United States; 2005. p. 1600–1602.

[48] Lombardo A, Rizzello V, Natale L, Lombardi M, Coli S, Snider F, Bonomo L, Crea F. Magnetic resonance imaging of carotid plaque inflammation in acute coronary syndromes: a sign of multisite plaque activation. *International journal of cardiology*. 2009 Jul 24;136(1):103-105.

[49] Choi S-H, Chae A, Chen C H, Merki E, Shaw P X, Tsimikas S. Emerging approaches for imaging vulnerable plaques in patients. *Curr. Opin. Biotechnol.* 2007 Feb;18(1):73–82.

[50] Abbate A, Bussani R, Liuzzo G, Biondi-Zoccai G G, Barresi E, Mellone P, Sinagra G, Dobrina A, De Giorgio F, Sharma R, Bassan F. Sudden coronary death, fatal

acute myocardial infarction and widespread coronary and myocardial inflammation. *Heart.* 2008 Jun 1;94(6):737-742.

[51] Doğan A, Kozan Ö, Tüzün N. Stent-içi restenozun fizyopatolojisi ve tedavisi (Physiopathology and treatment of intra-stent restenosis) *Türk Kardiyoloji Derneği Arşivi*. 2005;33(2):115-125.

[52] Dangas G D, Claessen B E, Caixeta A, Sanidas EA, Mintz GS, Mehran R. In-stent restenosis in the drug-eluting stent era. *J Am. .Coll. Cardiol.* 2010 Nov 30;56(23): 1897–907.

[53] Knudtson M L, Flintoft V F, Roth D L, Hansen J L, Duff H J. Effect of short-term prostacyclin administration on restenosis after percutaneous transluminal coronary angioplasty. *J. Am. Coll. Cardiol.* 1990 Mar 1;15(3):691–7.

[54] Kornowski R, Hong M K, Tio F O, Bramwell O, Wu H, Leon M B. In-stent restenosis: contributions of inflammatory responses and arterial injury to neointimal hyperplasia. *J. Am. Coll. Cardiol.* 1998 Jan;31(1):224–30.

[55] Bennett MR. In-stent stenosis: pathology and implications for the development of drug eluting stents. *Heart.* 2003 Feb;89(2):218–24.

[56] Lowe HC, Oesterle SN, Khachigian LM. Coronary in-stent restenosis: current status and future strategies. *J Am Coll Cardiol.* 2002 Jan;39(2):183–93.

[57] Mitchell RN, Libby P. Vascular remodeling in transplant vasculopathy. *Circ. Res.* 2007 Apr;100(7):967–78.

[58] Loeys B L, Schwarze U, Holm T, Callewaert BL, Thomas GH, Pannu H, De Backer JF, Oswald GL, Symoens S, Manouvrier S, Roberts AE. Aneurysm syndromes caused by mutations in the TGF-β receptor. *New England Journal of Medicine*. 2006 Aug 24;355(8):788-798.

[59] Alexander R W. Theodore Cooper Memorial Lecture. Hypertension and the pathogenesis of atherosclerosis. Oxidative stress and the mediation of arterial inflammatory response: a new perspective. *Hypertens.* 1995 Feb;25(2):155–161.

[60] Lüscher T F, Vanhoutte P M. Endothelium-dependent contractions to acetylcholine in the aorta of the spontaneously hypertensive rat. *Hypertens.* 1986 Apr;8(4):344–8.

[61] Ul Haq A, Carotenuto F, Di Nardo P, Francini R, Prosposito P, Pescosolido F, De Matteis F. Extrinsically conductive nanomaterials for cardiac tissue engineering applications. *Micromachines.* 2021 Jul 31;12(8):914.

[62] Rouwkema J, Khademhosseini A. Vascularization and Angiogenesis in Tissue Engineering: Beyond Creating Static Networks. *Trends Biotechnol.* 2016 Sep;34(9): 733–45.

[63] Wystrychowski W, Cierpka L, Zagalski K, Garrido S, Dusserre N, Radochonski S, McAllister TN, L'heureux N. Case study: first implantation of a frozen, devitalized tissue-engineered vascular graft for urgent hemodialysis access. *The journal of vascular access.* 2011 Jan;12(1):67-70.

Chapter 7

The Effect of Vascular Function on the Musculoskeletal System

Mehmet Ali Dursun*
Vakfikebir State Hospital, Department of Orthopaedics and Traumatology, Trabzon, Turkey

Abstract

The endothelium is an excellent barrier between the circulating blood and the vessel wall. It is considered the largest endocrine organ in the body, with the molecules it secretes and its receptors. The smooth functioning of the endothelium's special functions is essential for the perfect functioning of human physiology.

In a healthy endothelium, vasodilator, anti-inflammatory, antithrombotic factors, and vasoconstrictor, inflammatory and prothrombotic factors work in balance. Events that disrupt this balance cause endothelial dysfunction. Endothelial dysfunction may result in vasoconstriction, thrombus formation, increased inflammatory events, and increased cell proliferation. Endothelial dysfunction has been associated with many diseases, mainly atherosclerosis.

Endothelial functions are essential in the physiopathology and treatment of musculoskeletal diseases. In addition, endothelial damage is the main problem in the pathology of diseases in many areas, such as muscle-tendon injuries, enthesitis, tendinopathies, fracture healing, and cartilage problems.

In many treatments, such as fracture healing, therapy of tendinopathies, and repair of cartilage defects, the goal should be to help vascular functions work correctly and to improve endothelin functions for tissue healing. A better understanding of musculoskeletal diseases has

* Corresponding Author's Email: drmehmetalidursun@gmail.com.

In: Vascularization and Its Role in Medicine and Tissue Engineering
Editors: Emre Bulbul and Murat Oguz Ozilhan
ISBN: 979-8-89113-041-8

led us to seek both the source of the problem and the solution at the endothelial level.

Keywords: endothelium, endothelial dysfunction, musculoskeletal diseases, fracture healing, tissue engineering

Introduction

Endothel

Thirty years ago, the endothelium was considered a simple membrane. However, after Furchgott found the effect of acetylcholine in blood vessels in 1980, and then Ludmer in 1986 revealed the paradoxical effect of acetylcholine in coronary vessels, studies on endothelium gained momentum [1, 2]. As a result, the endothelium is considered a highly functional barrier consisting of endothelial cells between the vessel wall and the circulating blood.

The essential functions of the endothelium are to control the exchange of substances between the blood and the surrounding tissues, to regulate the balance of intravascular thrombosis and thrombolysis, and to regulate inflammation, immune response, and cell proliferation. The endothelium fulfils these tasks with the autocrine and paracrine secretions it secretes and many receptors on it [3].

In a healthy endothelium, vasodilator, anti-inflammatory, antithrombotic factors, and vasoconstrictor, inflammatory and prothrombotic factors work in balance. Events that disrupt this balance cause endothelial dysfunction. Endothelial dysfunction may result in vasoconstriction, thrombus formation, increased inflammatory events, and increased cell proliferation [4]. Endothelial dysfunction is considered a systemic disease, and many studies are being conducted on its early diagnosis, risk factors, and associated conditions [5].

The endothelium maintains the arrangement between vasodilation and vasoconstriction thanks to some molecules it produces and receptors on its surface. Nitric oxide (NO) produced from arginine by nitric oxide synthase (NOS) is the most potent vasodilation agent. It is also known as an endothelium-derived relaxing factor (EDRF). NO inhibits platelet aggregation, leukocyte adhesion, and excessive cell proliferation [6]. NO is converted to peroxynitrite (OONO-) by the enzyme superoxide dismutase in the presence of free oxygen radicals. Peroxynitrite is a highly potent oxidant substance and can cause genetic material damage within the cell [7, 8]. The most potent vasoconstrictors secreted by endothelin are endothelin and angiotensin II. In a healthy endothelium, vasoconstrictors and vasodilators work in balance. In conditions where production at the endothelial level and bioavailability in the cell will deteriorate, atherosclerosis and endothelial dysfunction, which can cause many diseases, occur in the clinic, starting with vasoconstriction, thrombosis, and increased inflammatory events [7, 9]. The first studies in this area were performed in coronary vessels occluded or decreased flow due to atherosclerosis. Finding that the vasodilation capacity and blood flow velocity of occluded vessels differs from those of healthy vessels has brought new studies.

Causes of Endothelial Dysfunction

Many different mechanisms have explained the cause of endothelial dysfunction. It has been stated that endothelial dysfunction occurs due to various abnormalities at the cellular and subcellular levels.

Disruption of the release balance and bioavailability of vasodilator and vasoconstrictor substances released from the endothelium is one of the most basic mechanisms. Nitric oxide is the most potent vasodilator released from the endothelium. NO produced by endothelial NOS inhibits platelet aggregation, neutrophil adhesion, and the production of other adhesion molecules and causes vasodilation by acting on smooth muscle cells. Oxygen radicals such as superoxide react with NO in the presence of superoxide dismutase and turn into radicals that are harmful to the cell, such as peroxynitrite [10].

It has been reported in the literature that many conditions, such as increased dietary fat, insulin intolerance, hypertension, smoking, obesity, increased androgen hormones, decreased physical activity, stress, menopause, reduced estrogen hormone, hereditary vascular diseases, hereditary glycogen, and fat storage diseases cause endothelial dysfunction. It has been suggested [11-13].

In the last ten years, molecular studies have been carried out to detect endothelial dysfunction in the early period, to prevent it from causing clinical problems in the long term, and to treat it at the cellular level. Research continues on the relationship between many issues such as magnesium deficiency, lack of antioxidant vitamins such as vitamins c and e, ionizing radiation effects, increased hemolysis, endoplasmic reticulum stress, tcrp3 channel mutations, increased concentration of oxygen radicals in the cell, lack of cofactors used in NO production, and endothelial dysfunction. [12, 14-17]. Although it has not been clarified whether clinically related diseases cause or consequence of endothelial dysfunction, it has been proven that endothelial dysfunction can ultimately result in atherosclerosis [13, 18].

Diagnostic Methods of Endothelial Dysfunction

Endothelial dysfunction is accepted as a systemic disease, and many studies have been conducted on its early diagnosis, risk factors, and associated conditions [19]. Recently, much work has been done with the thought that recognizing endothelial dysfunction can effectively manage and treat related conditions.

Serum markers, urinary metabolites, coronary studies, concurrent coronary studies with positron emission tomography, and invasive and noninvasive methods in peripheral vessels have revealed many options for diagnosing endothelial dysfunction. Current diagnostic methods for endothelial dysfunction are summarized in Table 1.

Table 1. Markers used in endothelial dysfunction

Author	Molecule	Year
Taddei	Endothelin 1	2001
Hlubocka	Endothelin 1, Icam, Vwf	2002
Faulx	Endothelin-1, Adma, Tpai, İcam, Vcam, E-Selectin, P-Selectin, Vwf	2003
Widlansky	Endothelin-1, İcam, Vcam, Tpai	2003
Horvath B.	Vwf	2004
Landmesser	Adma	2005
Thuillez	Endothelin 1	2005
Iglarz	Endothelin 1	2007
Deanfield	Adma, E-Selectin, P-Selectin, Vwf	2007
Münzel	Adma, E-Selectin, Vcam, Vwf, Crp, Epc.	2008
Ghiadoni	Adma, Epc	2008
Pericleous	Cd 133, Endothelial Microparticles	2009
Alba	EPC	2012
Cahill	Endothelin 1	2016
Agostini	Vwf	2017
Gawrys	Endothelin-1	2018

Abbreviations: Adma: asymmetric dimethyl arginine, Epc: endothelial progenitor cell, Icam: intravascular cell adhesion molecule, Tpai: tissue plasminogen activator inhibitor, Vcam: vascular cell adhesion molecule, vwf: von Willebrand factor.

Immediately after the definition of endothelial dysfunction, it was debated whether it would be a relevant marker in peripheral blood. However, there are many molecules in plasma that can be used in the diagnosis of endothelial dysfunction. These molecules' studies are in Table 2 [9-11, 19-30].

Table 2. The molecules used for the diagnosis of endothelial dysfunction in plasma

Serum markers	
*Endothelin-1 (ET-1), *Asymmetric dimethyl arginine (ADMA), *Von Willebrand factor (vWF), *Tissue plasminogen activator (t-PA),*Plasminogen activator inhibitor-1 (PAI-1), *Intercellular adhesion molecule (ICAMs), *Vascular cell adhesion molecule (VCAMs), *E-selectin, *P-selectin, *Endothelial progenitor cells (EPC), *Endothelial microparticles (CD133 etc.)	
Measurement of urinary metabolites	
*Measurement of nitric oxide and its metabolites in urine	
Coronary vascular studies	
Coronary studies with coronary angiography, positron emission tomography	
Peripheral vascular studies	
*Flow-mediated dilation method *Pulse wave curve method *Microvascular flow measurement with skin laser Doppler *Forearm/digital artery plethysmography with B2 agonist *Reactive hyperemia measurement with EndoPAT	Noninvasive methods
*Provocative functional tests in peripheral arteries *Brachial, radial, femoral artery plethysmography	Invasive methods

Peripheral Vascular Studies

Peripheral vascular studies started with the observation of Fleisch in 935, and then Heistad, Abboud, and Eckstein at different times that peripheral vessels respond to some stimuli by expanding or contracting [31, 32]. Finally, in 1986, Ludmer saw that the vasodilation response and flow amounts of healthy and occluded vessels were different due to the application of acetylcholine to the coronary arteries. Furthermore, he observed that while healthy vessels enlarge due to acetylcholine application, occluded vessels respond by contracting acetylcholine paradoxically. He associated this situation with the property of the vessel wall, and studies on the functions of endothelin started from this point.

These procedures were based on giving substances such as acetylcholine to the coronary vessels and looking at the amount of flow and their ability to expand, which were the main factors limiting the measurement. In addition, the high morbidity and mortality in coronary artery studies have led researchers to conduct similar studies on peripheral vessels.

Flow-Mediated Dilatation Method

In 1989, Anderson pioneered flow-mediated dilatation by showing that peripheral vessels can contract and expand independently of systemic pressure in the face of stress in his study on the brachial artery [33]. Over the following years, Celermajer and many researchers have developed a method allowing noninvasive flow-mediated dilatation measurement [34].

The primary mechanism of flow-induced dilatation (USA) is the expansion of the lumen, mainly by nitric oxide released from the endothelium, in response to the stress encountered by the vessel wall. This method also works on this principle and examines the stress response of the artificially stressed vessel wall. Flow-induced dilatation is mainly by endothelial NO and partially by prostacyclin, etc. It is considered to be mediated by vasodilators.

Endothelial function is evaluated by calculating the difference between the vessel lumen diameter measured using ultrasonography before and after stress. Technically, the measurement is made 5-10 centimeters (cm) above the cubital fossa using 7.5 Mhz or 12 Mhz linear probes, ideally accompanied by electrocardiography (ECG). Most commonly, the cuff is placed proximal to the forearm. At the end of the diastole of the brachial artery, just before the onset of the P wave, the distance between the anterior and posterior lumen diameters is measured by longitudinal sections and recorded as the basal diameter value. This process is repeated 3-5 times, and the arithmetic average of the measured basal diameter is recorded. Then, the cuff placed on the forearm is inflated 50 mmHg above the systolic blood pressure or up to 250-300 mmHg, and measurements are resumed while the cuff is abruptly lowered after 5 minutes of ischemia. The size is made by recording for 2 minutes. At the end of the test, the arterial diameter at the moment the flow-related dilatation is most significant is recorded (usually 60 seconds). The difference between the most dilatation value and the basal diameter value is calculated, and how much the result changes in the basal measurement is calculated by summing the percentage. This value is expressed as the endothelial function.

Nitrate Dependent Dilation Method

As described by Celermajer, ten minutes after cuff deflating, the patient is given 0.4 mg of sublingual/spray nitroglycerin (NTG) unless contraindicated. After NTG, the maximum dilatation value is measured again, which is 3-4 minutes, the time reported with the most dilatation. The value calculated after nitroglycerin is endothelium-independent flow-mediated dilatation (NBD: nitrate-induced dilatation). While the cut-off value of endothelial dysfunction has been found differently in different studies in the literature, the 10% change value is the most accepted limit. As a result, less than 10% response to stress is interpreted as endothelial dysfunction.

It is the most recommended flow-mediated dilatation method among endothelial dysfunction diagnostic methods in terms of noninvasive, inexpensive, reproducibility, specificity, and specificity (Figure 1). In addition, although this method can be performed on both the arm and the forearm, the brachial artery flow-related dilatation measurement technique is the most preferred in terms of ease of operation (Figure 2).

The Effect of the Vascular Function on the Musculoskeletal System

Endothelial functions are essential in the physiopathology and treatment of musculoskeletal diseases. Endothelial damage is the main problem in the pathology of diseases in many areas, such as muscle-tendon injuries, enthesitis, tendinopathies, fracture healing, and cartilage problems. Therefore, in many treatments, such as fracture healing, therapy of tendinopathies, and repair of cartilage defects, the goal should be to help vascular functions work correctly and to improve endothelial functions for tissue healing.

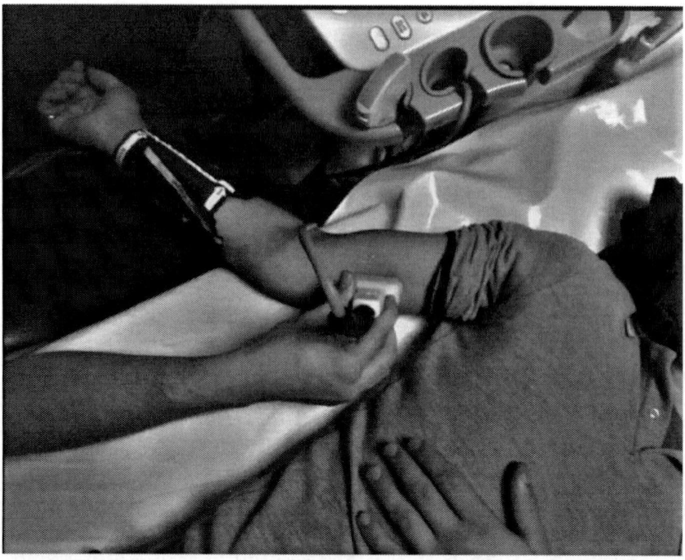

Figure 1. Endothelial function measurement of a patient in our clinic with the flow-mediated dilation technique.

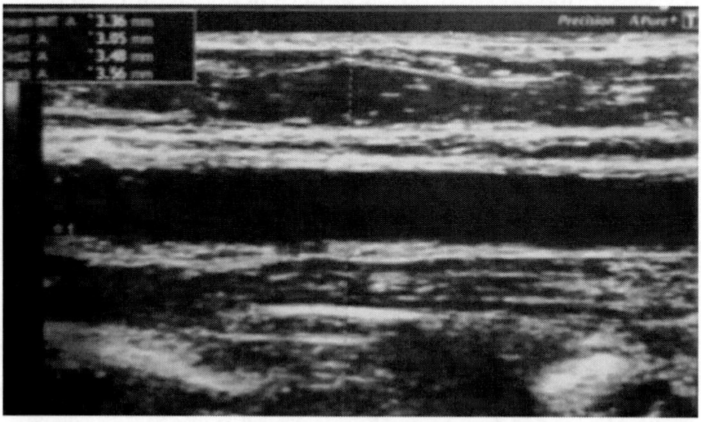

Figure 2. Ultrasonography image of the flow-mediated dilation technique performed in our clinic.

Fracture Healing

The first cellular response to tissue damage is inflammation. Inflammation includes a series of reactions caused by tissue damage and all the processes necessary for repair. Inflammation can be acute or chronic. Acute inflammation is the most common type. Initially, neutrophils migrate to the damaged area, and the endothelium releases secretions that increase endothelial permeability. The aim is to ensure the transition of proteins in the plasma to the site of inflammation. In this way, the repair mechanism functions.

When the anatomical structure is disrupted in bone or soft tissue, for example, due to a bone fracture, the endosteum, periosteum, and surrounding soft tissues are damaged. Meanwhile, blood and lymphatic vessels are also fragmented, and blood, lymph fluid, and exudate accumulate between tissues; this is called fracture hematoma.

Fracture hematoma is the source of hematopoietic cells that release bone growth factors and mesenchymal cells that differentiate and provide fracture healing. In addition, platelets in the fracture hematoma and other cells in the environment; secrete growth factors and necessary proteins. These factors and proteins are required for cell migration, periosteal cell proliferation, and synthesis of repair tissue matrix, which are essential in fracture healing. Due to post-fracture vasodilation and concomitant plasma exudation, edema occurs at the fracture site within the first 24 hours. Acute inflammation cells, especially leukocytes, migrate to the area. The hematoma in the fracture area is organized within 48 hours and forms a fibrinous structure. The fibrin matrix is formed by the extravasation of polymorph-nucleated leukocytes and macrophages, and cell proliferation, which is necessary for bone formation, begins. Stimuli that initiate fracture repair are probably chemotactic factors released at the fracture site during inflammation and matrix proteins released by bone tissue fragmentation. Cells involved in the repair process are pluripotent cells of mesenchymal origin.

Mesenchymal cells at the fracture site proliferate and differentiate to form what is known as the 'fracture callus,' which contains fibrous tissue, cartilage, and lattice bone. A granulation tissue develops by the proliferation and differentiation of periosteal and endosteal osteogenic cells and fibroblasts in the fibrin matrix. Towards the end of the first week, islands of cartilage appear in the granulation tissue that replaces the hematoma. After this stage, the mineralization stage requires the formation of the necessary conditions to heal the fracture. Essential conditions for adequate mineralization; Sufficient concentration of calcium and phosphate ions, the matrix that can be calcified, matrix vesicles, and collagen are the control of regulatory factors. In this stage, ossification arrest leads to pseudoarthrosis, known as nonunion or pseudarthrosis. Typical findings are pause at this stage, mineralization and vascularization disruption, the union's absence, and delayed union [35]. The mineralization of the osteoid is necessary for the formation of hard callus and structural stability. Callus: It occurs more slowly in adults than in children, and more slowly in compact bone than in trabecular bone. In the middle of the repair phase, remodeling begins with the reabsorption of redundant parts of the callus and the extension of the trabecular bone along the stress lines. While the remodeling phase in adults takes years, it occurs quite quickly in children. From the moment the fracture occurs, different amounts of fracture hematoma and healing tissue appear, depending on the type of fracture (open fracture, closed fracture) and the amount of energy. In other words, the body transfers the substances necessary for the healing of the fracture to the fracture site with local or systemic sources. At the same time, it tries to increase blood flow and neural transmission to the fracture site, if possible. When the fracture occurs, multipotent cells grow both in the fracture site and the circulation, stimulating the receptors to secrete the factors necessary for fracture healing. The primary mechanism in vascular diseases such as occlusive vascular diseases, kidney failure, smoking, hypertension, and diabetes is atherosclerosis, starting from small arteries and developing up to large main arteries. Due to atherosclerosis, the small vessels cannot provide blood flow, and the substances necessary for bone healing will hardly or may not reach the fracture site. As a result, fracture healing will be delayed or absent in chronic diseases in which vascular functions are impaired [36].

Nonunion

In cases where fracture healing does not occur despite waiting for sufficient time, traumatologists investigate why the fracture does not heal. As a result of clinical and radiological evaluations, fracture healing is differentiated as atrophic nonunion and hypertrophic nonunion [37]. In the type where the vascular supply of the fracture line is good, there are enough tissues in the fracture area, but the fracture does not union due to lack of fixation. The type in which vascular nutrition is not good at the fracture line is atrophic nonunion. This type of nonunion consists for different reasons in itself. Due to the anatomical structure of the bone, in cases where the fracture line disrupts nutrition (proximal scaphoid fractures, femur neck fractures, talus fractures), soft tissue damage caused by fracture energy, and open fractures in which the vascular structures are damaged, the fracture area cannot be adequately nourished, and atrophic nonunion occurs [38, 39].

The first aim of treating atrophic nonunions with insufficient nutrition is to get the area bloody. Decortication of the fracture line, bone marrow stimulation methods applied to the fracture line, autogenous bone graft transplants, and vascular bone graft applications have been developed and successfully used in the treatment. In cases where nonunion does not occur despite all treatments, bone integrity is achieved by segment shifting or lengthening treatment with external fixators.

Ilizarov Method

Posttraumatic, infectious nonunion of long bones or congenital or acquired shortness and deformities are still problems that are difficult to treat. Various treatment principles such as Papineau-type open grafting, fibula-pro-tibia, and internal or external have been applied, but these techniques have high complication rates. In addition, in these old methods, fundamental problems such as local osteoporosis occurring in the extremity due to long-term non-weight bearing decreased blood circulation and inability to eliminate the shortness difference arise.

In the limb lengthening techniques, which started in the early 1900s, a new era opened with the method developed by Ilizarov in 1950. In his experiments on dogs, Ilizarov described a technique in which taut wires, passed over the skin to the proximal and distal ends of the bone, are tightly fixed with rings after osteotomy on long bones with a particular principle. Distraction or compression can occur at the fracture line by connecting the proximal and distal rings with a portable system [40]. As a result of his long experiments, Ilizarov explained how the lengthening of the bone occurs in the closest way to physiology. According to the technique, 1 mm lengthening per day has been described as a result of 0.25 mm distraction performed at the fracture ends every six hours. In the first stage of the Ilizarov technique, the broken ends are compressed together. The compression period averages seven days. At the end of this period, the distraction phase can start without waiting or waiting for seven days [41]. In the Ilizarov method, regional blood flow is increased after resuscitation of the fracture ends or osteotomy of the intact bone. Increasing inflammation and blood flow allow multipotent cells to reach the region in the first stage. At the same time, if the method is applied to cause infectious nonunion, increased blood flow is an essential advantage for treatment. With the onset of distraction, osteoblastic activity begins to increase ideally. Local blood flow increases, and new collaterals form that feed the area. Just as in the stages of callus formation, the bone tissue formed by osteoblastic activity is first remodelled after the mineralization of cartilage islands and osteoid and takes its final form. Ilizarov perfectly explained this with his experiments. He described the frequency of 1 mm of distraction per day according to the histochemical development of all soft tissues around the arterioles, smooth muscles, and bone. As a result, he stated that 0.17 mm of distraction performed once in 24 minutes by the auto-distractor may be the best for lengthening soft tissues and bone tissue [42].

The Ilizarov technique has been developed with modern devices, and the complication rate has been minimized. From the first moment, patients continue their lives by giving a load. In addition, the instruments used have decreased in size, and patient comfort has increased considerably. Recently, extensions made using externally controlled systems with nails and magnetic receivers, all of which are in the bone, are the most frequently used implants.

Avascular Necrosis

Its cartilage type 2 collagen-weighted structure has a smooth anatomical structure that provides movement and lubrication on the joint surfaces. The subchondral bone just below the cartilage tissue and the metaphyseal bone tissue beneath it are the supporting tissues of the cartilage surface. While bone provides tissue nutrition directly from the vascular structures with blood flow, cartilage is fed from the joint and subchondral bone by diffusion. Anatomical defects in the subchondral bone can now cause damage to the cartilage structure. The blood supply disorder in the subchondral bone causes avascular necrosis in cartilage. When avascular necrosis occurs, the microarchitecture and then the morphology of the cartilage tissue deteriorates, and a non-load-bearing, pressure-sensitive, smooth surface deteriorates tissue. This situation, which causes pain and limitation of movement in the clinic, constitutes 10 percent of arthroplasty cases. Many factors are involved in the etiology of avascular necrosis. The most common causes are trauma, idiopathic, occlusive vascular diseases, alcohol, steroid use, and autoimmune diseases [43].

The most commonly known cause of avascular necrosis is the underlying blood supply disorder. The explanation for many conditions, such as damage to the vessels feeding the subchondral bone due to trauma, occlusive vascular diseases, autoimmune diseases, and steroid use, is the deterioration of the blood supply to the bone tissue under the cartilage. In the subchondral bone, whose blood supply is impaired, edema and inflammation develop first. At this stage, at the beginning of the disease, there is no pain in the clinic, no X-ray finding, and only edema is present in the MRI. As the inflammation in the bone tissue increases, the exchange of cells with the extracellular matrix begins to deteriorate. Cell necrosis begins to appear. At this stage, loss of touch begins to form in the subchondral bone. X-ray shows subchondral bone cysts and sclerosis. As the disease progresses, bone tissue loss spreads over a wider area, and the subchondral bone collapses. The condition is now advanced.

After this stage, the articular surface deteriorates, and arthritis develops. In the final stages, the disease becomes irreversible. Although the treatment of avascular necrosis varies according to the joint and age, in general, the first treatments begin with load restriction, rest, and analgesics. After that, conservative treatment includes bisphosphonate, hyperbaric oxygen therapy, anticoagulant use, and statin use, which do not yet have a high level of evidence [44]. The primary purpose of statin therapy is to help improve vascular functions by balancing blood lipid levels [45].

Hyperbaric oxygen therapy contributes to nitric oxide metabolism by preventing hypoxia and increasing antioxidant production. In this way, it is predicted that both tissue oxygenation will increase and vascular functions will improve. In cases where conservative treatment fails, surgical methods include core decompression, bone-cartilage tissue transfers with vascular flaps, angled osteotomies, and arthroplasties [46].

Enthesitis-Tendinopathies

The most common problems encountered by orthopedists in the clinic are issues in the tendon-bone junction, such as plantar fasciitis, lateral epicondylitis, rotator cuff tendinopathy, and Achilles tendinopathy. The most common etiology of these diseases is overuse, repetitive movements, and occupational exposures [47]. If we look at the common pathophysiology of the conditions, it is striking that there are problems in the region of attachment of the tendons closest to the bone. Most microscopic damage in these insertion zones, the avascular zone or the hypovascular zone, can be healed with rest and a suitable repair mechanism. However, continuous activity or similar movements do not make this recovery possible in some people. Continuing inflammation prevents a smooth transition to the repair phase, and ultimately painful and defective movements occur [48].

Microvascular thrombosis is thought to be the underlying pathophysiology of these diseases. As a result, thrombosis in small vascular beds prevents adequate vascular nutrition in the inflammation area. As a result, chronic inflammation continues, but the repair phase cannot occur.

Rest, assistive devices such as braces and braces, rehabilitation protocols such as stretching exercises, and anti-inflammatory analgesic agents are used to treat these diseases. In most cases, conservative treatment works, but some patients fail this treatment. In these cases, some treatments come to the fore to increase the area's blood supply. For example, in lateral epicondylitis, the purpose of the decortication of the periosteum by the injector in the injections made to the elbow and the decortication applied to the ligament adhesion site in plantar fasciitis is to increase the blood supply to the periosteum and to provide growth factors from the subchondral bone to the region to provide healing.

Different techniques are applied to the attachment points of the torn tendon in rotator sheath repair, to the degenerated parts of the torn ends in meniscal tears, and to the ruptured tendon ends in tendon repairs while an end-to-end repair is performed. These techniques, which are recommended in standard methods, are decortication applied to the attachment sites, and the degenerative parts of the areas to be repaired are excised and vascularized. Adequate vascular nutrition is possible by reaching the bleeding tissues during surgery; thus, the necessary conditions for recovery will be provided.

Tissue Engineering

Anatomical disorders in the musculoskeletal system often heal almost entirely without loss of function under physiological conditions—one of the most critical factors in the traditional methods applied in the absence of tissue defect. However, when bone or connective tissue is damaged, the incomplete healing mechanism in the injury area or tissue loss in the damaged area fails healing and necrosis of the damaged area in most cases. In this case, the treatment to be applied should be to place scaffold frameworks, autogenous or allogeneous grafts, and synthetic materials that mimic the tissue and stimulate cell migration for support, after the cavity is cleaned and becomes a bloody area. In short, the aim is to place the material in the hole, stimulating the necessary mechanism for healing, providing migration to the region, and providing a suitable ground for new tissue formation. With these materials, treatments that stimulate healing, such as Platelet Rich Plasma, can be applied to the area.

Platelet Rich Plasma

One of the treatments used in musculoskeletal diseases is the platelet-rich plasma (PRP) procedure, which has become increasingly common in recent years [49]. PRP is obtaining high-density platelet-containing plasma in different forms after centrifuging the blood from the person's body under certain conditions. PRP is essentially a fluid containing dense platelets. Alpha, dense, and gamma granules are located in the platelets. Alpha granules contain growth factors and cytokines. Gamma granules contain serotonin, polyphosphates, calcium, and adenosine triphosphate.

Among the growth factors in alpha granules, fibroblast growth factor-2(FGF-2), platelet-derived growth factor (PDGF), tissue growth factor b(TGF-b), vascular endothelial growth factor (VEGF), and insulin-like growth factor (IGF) exist [50]. VEGF increases vascular permeability and contributes to vascular hyperplasia and mitogenic activity. PDGF increases mitogenic activity and provides cell differentiation. FGF aids chemotaxis and suppresses macrophage and lymphocyte activity. In addition, it is involved in producing collagen in bone and muscle tissue. IGF increases mitogenic activity in osteoblast production and helps chemotactic activities. PRP also contains cytokines. Cytokines and growth factors, which have essential roles in tissue healing, play a role in cell chemotaxis, cell proliferation, and differentiation. PRP contains essential cytokines such as interleukin-1 (IL-1b) and tumor necrosis factor-a (TNF-a). IL-1b and TNF-a nuclear factor-B (NF-kB) are essential in controlling inflammation by activating the signaling pathway.

Thanks to the intense growth factors and cytokines in PRP, it provides early vascularization and contributes to tissue healing. In the PRP musculoskeletal system, which has been used in many areas recently, the recommended usage areas are generally fracture healing, muscle-tendon injuries, tendinopathies, peripheral nerve injuries, non-healing wounds, and treatment of osteochondral lesions. PRP therapy can be used as adjunctive therapy when fracture healing does not occur or is delayed. The growth factors and cytokines contained in it will stimulate healing, and at the same time, osteoblast production will accelerate by promoting cell differentiation and increasing vascularization. Mesenchymal stem cells (MSCs) accelerate bone morphological protein-2 production, and osteoinductive capacity increases. PRP application to the recipient site and autogenous bone graft has been accepted most frequently in the clinic [51].

Muscle-tendon injuries are problems that orthopedists frequently encounter in daily practice, especially concerning sports injuries. They are considered acute or chronic. They usually occur due to the construction of repetitive movements or compulsive movements. Healing of muscle fiber injuries is generally uneventful. In contrast, injuries to the muscle-tendon junction or tendon area are often difficult to treat due to the anatomically poor blood supply to these areas. In incomplete recovery cases, chronic pain, weakness, limitation in activities, and incomplete return to sports are seen. Tendon regeneration is accelerated by stimulating Tendon stem cells and cell differentiation in PRP. Kim et al. stated that combining bone marrow and PRP in patients with rotator cuff tendinopathy accelerated healing [52]. In another study, Zhang et al. said that tendon regeneration would be faster after PRP application, which is rich in leukocytes. More cell differentiation was observed compared to pure PRP application [53]. Li et al. showed that TGF-B in PRP content reduced healing without fibrosis after PRP application [54].

Peripheral nerve injuries may occur due to trauma, tourniquet, infectious diseases, autoimmune diseases, and idiopathic causes. Nerve damage can range from mild neuropraxia to complete loss of conduction. This axonal damage is often directly proportional to its severity. The regeneration capacity in nervous tissue is quite limited compared to other tissues [55]. In open fractures, the gold standard is nerve repair in nerve cuts due to the mechanism of injury and grafting of the nerve in late cases [56]. It is suggested that applying PRP with this technique increases the regeneration capacity. Abundant growth factors and cytokines in PRP may promote successful repair by accelerating Schwann cell activation, early vascularization, fibrogenesis, angiogenesis, and macrophage polarization [57]. PRP may also work as support tissue for neuroregeneration [58].

Conclusion

A better understanding of musculoskeletal diseases has led us to seek both the source of the problem and the solution at the endothelial level. With the developing technology and time gaining value, efforts are being made to improve musculoskeletal problems faster. Supportive treatments to shorten the physiological recovery period are gradually developing, and the cost is increasing in this area. Nevertheless, significant gains have been achieved in the last ten years in muscle-tendon problems, and treatment times have shortened considerably. We think that in the future, these problems will be better understood, and treatments that will regulate and significantly accelerate the functioning of cellular and subcellular mechanisms will come to the fore.

References

[1] Furchgott RF, Zawadzki JV. The obligatory role of endothelial cells in the relaxation of arterial smooth muscle by acetylcholine. *Nature.* 1980 Nov 27;288(5789):373-6. doi: 10.1038/288373a0. PMID: 6253831.

[2] Ludmer PL, Selwyn AP, Shook TL, Wayne RR, Mudge GH, Alexander RW, Ganz P. Paradoxical vasoconstriction induced by acetylcholine in atherosclerotic coronary arteries. *N Engl J Med.* 1986 Oct 23;315(17):1046-51. doi: 10.1056/NEJM198610233151702. PMID: 3093861.

[3] Celermajer DS. Endothelial dysfunction: does it matter? Is it reversible? *J Am Coll Cardiol.* 1997 Aug;30(2):325-33. doi: 10.1016/s0735-1097(97)00189-7. PMID: 9247501.

[4] Poredos P. Endothelial dysfunction in the pathogenesis of atherosclerosis. *Clin Appl Thromb Hemost.* 2001 Oct;7(4):276-80. doi: 10.1177/107602960100700404. PMID: 11697708.

[5] Anderson TJ. Assessment and treatment of endothelial dysfunction in humans. *J Am Coll Cardiol.* 1999 Sep;34(3):631-8. doi: 10.1016/s0735-1097(99)00259-4. PMID: 10483941.

[6] Kubes P, Suzuki M, Granger DN. Nitric oxide: an endogenous modulator of leukocyte adhesion. *Proc Natl Acad Sci U S A.* 1991 Jun 1;88(11):4651-5. doi: 10.1073/pnas.88.11.4651. PMID: 1675786; PMCID: PMC51723.

[7] Le Brocq M, Leslie SJ, Milliken P, Megson IL. Endothelial dysfunction: from molecular mechanisms to measurement, clinical implications, and therapeutic opportunities. *Antioxid Redox Signal.* 2008 Sep;10(9):1631-74. doi: 10.1089/ars.2007.2013. PMID: 18598143.

[8] Godo S, Shimokawa H. Endothelial Functions. *Arterioscler Thromb Vasc Biol.* 2017 Sep;37(9):e108-e114. doi: 10.1161/ATVBAHA.117.309813. PMID: 28835487.

[9] Deanfield JE, Halcox JP, Rabelink TJ. Endothelial function and dysfunction: testing and clinical relevance. *Circulation.* 2007 Mar 13;115(10):1285-95. doi: 10.1161/CIRCULATIONAHA.106.652859. PMID: 17353456.

[10] Münzel T, Sinning C, Post F, Warnholtz A, Schulz E. Pathophysiology, diagnosis and prognostic implications of endothelial dysfunction. *Ann Med.* 2008;40(3):180-96. doi: 10.1080/07853890701854702. PMID: 18382884.

[11] Cahill PA, Redmond EM. Vascular endothelium - Gatekeeper of vessel health. *Atherosclerosis.* 2016 May;248:97-109. doi: 10.1016/j.atherosclerosis.2016.03.007. Epub 2016 Mar 9. PMID: 26994427; PMCID: PMC6478391.

[12] Maamoun H, Abdelsalam SS, Zeidan A, Korashy HM, Agouni A. Endoplasmic Reticulum Stress: A Critical Molecular Driver of Endothelial Dysfunction and Cardiovascular Disturbances Associated with Diabetes. *Int J Mol Sci.* 2019 Apr 3;20(7):1658. doi: 10.3390/ijms20071658. PMID: 30987118; PMCID: PMC6480154.

[13] Bonetti PO, Lerman LO, Lerman A. Endothelial dysfunction: a marker of atherosclerotic risk. *Arterioscler Thromb Vasc Biol.* 2003 Feb 1;23(2):168-75. doi: 10.1161/01.atv.0000051384.43104.fc. PMID: 12588755.

[14] Smedlund K, Bah M, Vazquez G. On the role of endothelial TRPC3 channels in endothelial dysfunction and cardiovascular disease. *Cardiovasc Hematol Agents Med Chem.* 2012 Sep;10(3):265-74. doi: 10.2174/187152512802651051. PMID: 22827251; PMCID: PMC3465809.

[15] Wolf FI, Trapani V, Simonacci M, Ferré S, Maier JA. Magnesium deficiency and endothelial dysfunction: is oxidative stress involved? *Magnes Res.* 2008 Mar;21(1):58-64. PMID: 18557135.

[16] Baselet B, Sonveaux P, Baatout S, Aerts A. Pathological effects of ionizing radiation: endothelial activation and dysfunction. *Cell Mol Life Sci.* 2019 Feb;76(4):699-728. doi: 10.1007/s00018-018-2956-z. Epub 2018 Oct 30. PMID: 30377700; PMCID: PMC6514067.

[17] Vinchi F, Tolosano E. Therapeutic approaches to limit hemolysis-driven endothelial dysfunction: scavenging free heme to preserve vasculature homeostasis. *Oxid Med Cell Longev.* 2013;2013:396527. doi: 10.1155/2013/396527. Epub 2013 May 27. PMID: 23781294; PMCID: PMC3678425.

[18] Ambrosino P, Lupoli R, Iervolino S, De Felice A, Pappone N, Storino A, Di Minno MND. Clinical assessment of endothelial function in patients with chronic obstructive pulmonary disease: a systematic review with meta-analysis. *Intern Emerg Med.* 2017 Sep;12(6):877-885. doi: 10.1007/s11739-017-1690-0. Epub 2017 Jun 7. PMID: 28593450.

[19] Landmesser U, Drexler H. The clinical significance of endothelial dysfunction. *Curr Opin Cardiol.* 2005 Nov;20(6):547-51. doi: 10.1097/01.hco.0000179821.11071.79. PMID: 16234629.

[20] Taddei S, Virdis A, Ghiadoni L, Sudano I, Salvetti A. Endothelial dysfunction in hypertension. *J Cardiovasc Pharmacol.* 2001 Nov;38 Suppl 2:S11-4. doi: 10.1097/00005344-200111002-00004. PMID: 11811368.

[21] Hlubocká Z, Umnerová V, Heller S, Peleska J, Jindra A, Jáchymová M, Kvasnicka J, Horký K, Aschermann M. Circulating intercellular cell adhesion molecule-1, endothelin-1 and von Willebrand factor-markers of endothelial dysfunction in uncomplicated essential hypertension: the effect of treatment with ACE inhibitors. *J Hum Hypertens.* 2002 Aug;16(8):557-62. doi: 10.1038/sj.jhh.1001403. PMID: 12149661.

[22] Faulx MD, Wright AT, Hoit BD. Detection of endothelial dysfunction with brachial artery ultrasound scanning. *Am Heart J.* 2003 Jun;145(6):943-51. doi: 10.1016/S0002-8703(03)00097-8. PMID: 12796748.

[23] Widlansky ME, Gokce N, Keaney JF Jr, Vita JA. The clinical implications of endothelial dysfunction. *J Am Coll Cardiol.* 2003 Oct 1;42(7):1149-60. doi: 10.1016/s0735-1097(03)00994-x. PMID: 14522472.

[24] Horvath B, Hegedus D, Szapary L, Marton Z, Alexy T, Koltai K, Czopf L, Wittmann I, Juricskay I, Toth K, Kesmarky G. Measurement of von Willebrand factor as the marker of endothelial dysfunction in vascular diseases. *Exp Clin Cardiol.* 2004 Spring;9(1):31-4. PMID: 19641694; PMCID: PMC2716260.

[25] Thuillez C, Richard V. Targeting endothelial dysfunction in hypertensive subjects. *J Hum Hypertens.* 2005 Jun;19 Suppl 1:S21-5. doi: 10.1038/sj.jhh.1001889. PMID: 16075029.

[26] Ghiadoni L, Versari D, Giannarelli C, Faita F, Taddei S. Non-invasive diagnostic tools for investigating endothelial dysfunction. *Curr Pharm Des.* 2008;14(35):3715-22. doi: 10.2174/138161208786898761. PMID: 19128224.

[27] Pericleous C, Giles I, Rahman A. Are endothelial microparticles potential markers of vascular dysfunction in the antiphospholipid syndrome? *Lupus.* 2009 Jul;18(8):671-5. doi: 10.1177/0961203309103062. PMID: 19502261.

[28] Alba AC, Delgado DH, Rao V, Walter S, Guyatt G, Ross HJ. Are endothelial progenitor cells a prognostic factor in patients with heart failure? *Expert Rev Cardiovasc Ther.* 2012 Feb;10(2):167-75. doi: 10.1586/erc.11.178. PMID: 22292873.

[29] Agostini S, Lionetti V. New insights into the non-hemostatic role of von Willebrand factor in endothelial protection. *Can J Physiol Pharmacol.* 2017 Oct;95(10):1183-1189. doi: 10.1139/cjpp-2017-0126. Epub 2017 Jul 17. PMID: 28715643.

[30] Gawrys J, Gawrys K, Szahidewicz-Krupska E, Derkacz A, Mochol J, Doroszko A. Interactions between the Cyclooxygenase Metabolic Pathway and the Renin-Angiotensin-Aldosterone Systems: Their Effect on Cardiovascular Risk, from Theory to the Clinical Practice. *Biomed Res Int.* 2018 Oct 2;2018:7902081. doi: 10.1155/2018/7902081. PMID: 30386795; PMCID: PMC6189683.

[31] Abboud FM, Eckstein JW. Comparative changes in segmental vascular resistance in response to nerve stimulation and to norepinephrine. *Circ Res.* 1966 Mar;18(3):263-77. doi: 10.1161/01.res.18.3.263. PMID: 5904317.

[32] Heistad DD, Abbound FM, Eckstein JW. Vasoconstrictor response to simulated diving in man. *J Appl Physiol.* 1968 Nov;25(5):542-9. doi: 10.1152/jappl.1968.25.5.542. PMID: 5687360.

[33] Anderson EA, Mark AL. Flow-mediated and reflex changes in large peripheral artery tone in humans. *Circulation.* 1989 Jan;79(1):93-100. doi: 10.1161/01.cir.79.1.93. PMID: 2910548.

[34] Celermajer DS, Sorensen KE, Gooch VM, Spiegelhalter DJ, Miller OI, Sullivan ID, Lloyd JK, Deanfield JE. Non-invasive detection of endothelial dysfunction in children and adults at risk of atherosclerosis. *Lancet.* 1992 Nov 7;340(8828):1111-5. doi: 10.1016/0140-6736(92)93147-f. PMID: 1359209.

[35] Zura R, Mehta S, Della Rocca GJ, Steen RG. Biological Risk Factors for Nonunion of Bone Fracture. *JBJS Rev.* 2016 Jan 5;4(1):e5. doi: 10.2106/JBJS.RVW.O.00008. PMID: 27490008.

[36] Hak DJ. Management of aseptic tibial nonunion. *J Am Acad Orthop Surg.* 2011 Sep;19(9):563-73. doi: 10.5435/00124635-201109000-00007. PMID: 21885702.

[37] Jones DB Jr, Bürger H, Bishop AT, Shin AY. Treatment of scaphoid waist nonunions with an avascular proximal pole and carpal collapse. A comparison of two vascularized bone grafts. *J Bone Joint Surg Am.* 2008 Dec;90(12):2616-25. doi: 10.2106/JBJS.G.01503. PMID: 19047706.

[38] Mathews V, Cabanela ME. Femoral neck nonunion treatment. *Clin Orthop Relat Res.* 2004 Feb;(419):57-64. doi: 10.1097/00003086-200402000-00010. PMID: 15021132.

[39] Bishop JA, Palanca AA, Bellino MJ, Lowenberg DW. Assessment of compromised fracture healing. *J Am Acad Orthop Surg.* 2012 May;20(5):273-82. doi: 10.5435/JAAOS-20-05-273. PMID: 22553099.

[40] Ilizarov GA. The tension-stress effect on the genesis and growth of tissues. Part I. The influence of stability of fixation and soft-tissue preservation. *Clin Orthop Relat Res.* 1989 Jan;(238):249-81. PMID: 2910611.

[41] Ilizarov GA. The tension-stress effect on the genesis and growth of tissues: Part II. The influence of the rate and frequency of distraction. *Clin Orthop Relat Res.* 1989 Feb;(239):263-85. PMID: 2912628.

[42] Ilizarov GA. Clinical application of the tension-stress effect for limb lengthening. *Clin Orthop Relat Res.* 1990 Jan;(250):8-26. PMID: 2403497.

[43] Zalavras CG, Lieberman JR. Osteonecrosis of the femoral head: evaluation and treatment. *J Am Acad Orthop Surg.* 2014 Jul;22(7):455-64. doi: 10.5435/JAAOS-22-07-455. PMID: 24966252.

[44] Lai KA, Shen WJ, Yang CY, Shao CJ, Hsu JT, Lin RM. The use of alendronate to prevent early collapse of the femoral head in patients with nontraumatic osteonecrosis. A randomized clinical study. *J Bone Joint Surg Am.* 2005 Oct;87(10): 2155-9. doi: 10.2106/JBJS.D.02959. PMID: 16203877.

[45] Tousoulis D, Papageorgiou N, Androulakis E, Paroutoglou K, Stefanadis C. Novel therapeutic strategies targeting vascular endothelium in essential hypertension. *Expert Opin Investig Drugs.* 2010 Nov;19(11):1395-412. doi: 10.1517/13543784.2010.522989. Epub 2010 Oct 5. PMID: 20923260.

[46] Cao L, Guo C, Chen J, Chen Z, Yan Z. Free Vascularized Fibular Grafting Improves Vascularity Compared With Core Decompression in Femoral Head Osteonecrosis: A Randomized Clinical Trial. *Clin Orthop Relat Res.* 2017 Sep;475(9):2230-2240. doi: 10.1007/s11999-017-5374-x. Epub 2017 May 4. PMID: 28474152; PMCID: PMC5539029.

[47] Calfee RP, Patel A, DaSilva MF, Akelman E. Management of lateral epicondylitis: current concepts. *J Am Acad Orthop Surg.* 2008 Jan;16(1):19-29. doi: 10.5435/00124635-200801000-00004. PMID: 18180389.

[48] Drake ML, Ring DC. Enthesopathy of the Extensor Carpi Radialis Brevis Origin: Effective Communication Strategies. *J Am Acad Orthop Surg.* 2016 Jun;24(6):365-9. doi: 10.5435/JAAOS-D-15-00233. PMID: 27077478.

[49] Mishra AK, Skrepnik NV, Edwards SG, Jones GL, Sampson S, Vermillion DA, Ramsey ML, Karli DC, Rettig AC. Efficacy of platelet-rich plasma for chronic tennis elbow: a double-blind, prospective, multicenter, randomized controlled trial

of 230 patients. *Am J Sports Med.* 2014 Feb;42(2):463-71. doi: 10.1177/03635465 13494359. Epub 2013 Jul 3. PMID: 23825183.

[50] Scully D, Naseem KM, Matsakas A. Platelet biology in regenerative medicine of skeletal muscle. *Acta Physiol* (Oxf). 2018 Jul;223(3):e13071. doi: 10.1111/ apha.13071. Epub 2018 Apr 19. PMID: 29633517.

[51] Krüger JP, Ketzmar AK, Endres M, Pruss A, Siclari A, Kaps C. Human platelet-rich plasma induces chondrogenic differentiation of subchondral progenitor cells in polyglycolic acid-hyaluronan scaffolds. *J Biomed Mater Res B Appl Biomater.* 2014 May;102(4):681-92. doi: 10.1002/jbm.b.33047. Epub 2013 Nov 26. PMID: 24510 445.

[52] Kim SJ, Song DH, Park JW, Park S, Kim SJ. Effect of Bone Marrow Aspirate Concentrate-Platelet-Rich Plasma on Tendon-Derived Stem Cells and Rotator Cuff Tendon Tear. *Cell Transplant.* 2017 May 9;26(5):867-878. doi: 10.3727/096368 917X694705. Epub 2017 Jan 20. PMID: 28105983; PMCID: PMC5657720.

[53] Zhang L, Chen S, Chang P, Bao N, Yang C, Ti Y, Zhou L, Zhao J. Harmful Effects of Leukocyte-Rich Platelet-Rich Plasma on Rabbit Tendon Stem Cells In Vitro. *Am J Sports Med.* 2016 Aug;44(8):1941-51. doi: 10.1177/0363546516644718. Epub 2016 May 16. PMID: 27184544.

[54] Li H, Hicks JJ, Wang L, Oyster N, Philippon MJ, Hurwitz S, Hogan MV, Huard J. Customized platelet-rich plasma with transforming growth factor β1 neutralization antibody to reduce fibrosis in skeletal muscle. *Biomaterials.* 2016 May;87:147-156. doi: 10.1016/j.biomaterials.2016.02.017. Epub 2016 Feb 17. PMID: 26923362.

[55] Zheng C, Zhu Q, Liu X, Huang X, He C, Jiang L, Quan D. Improved peripheral nerve regeneration using acellular nerve allografts loaded with platelet-rich plasma. *Tissue Eng Part A.* 2014 Dec;20(23-24):3228-40. doi: 10.1089/ten.TEA.2013.0729. PMID: 24901030; PMCID: PMC4259182.

[56] Bayram B, Akdeniz SS, Diker N, Helvacioğlu F, Erdem SR. Effects of Platelet-Rich Fibrin Membrane on Sciatic Nerve Regeneration. *J Craniofac Surg.* 2018 May;29(3):e239-e243. doi: 10.1097/SCS.0000000000004256. PMID: 29381631.

[57] Safa, B., Buncke, G. Autograft substitutes. Hand Clin 32, 127, 2016. Safa B, Buncke G. Autograft Substitutes: Conduits and Processed Nerve Allografts. *Hand Clin.* 2016 May;32(2):127-40. doi: 10.1016/j.hcl.2015.12.012. PMID: 27094886.

[58] Baklaushev VP, Bogush VG, Kalsin VA, Sovetnikov NN, Samoilova EM, Revkova VA, Sidoruk KV, Konoplyannikov MA, Timashev PS, Kotova SL, Yushkov KB, Averyanov AV, Troitskiy AV, Ahlfors JE. Tissue Engineered Neural Constructs Composed of Neural Precursor Cells, Recombinant Spidroin and PRP for Neural Tissue Regeneration. *Sci Rep.* 2019 Feb 28;9(1):3161. doi: 10.1038/s41598-019-39341-9. PMID: 30816182; PMCID: PMC6395623.

Chapter 8

Angiogenic Therapies, Tissue Implantations and Tissue Engineering in Urology

Emre Bulbul[1,*], MD
and Yavuz Ilki[2,†], MD
[1]Trabzon Vakfikebir State Hospital, Department of Urology, Trabzon, Turkey
[2]Gulhane Training and Research Hospital, Department of Urology, Ankara, Turkey

Abstract

Many treatment methods are being developed in modern medicine with innovative approaches. For example, regenerative therapies and tissue engineering are used in many fields of medicine. Regenerative therapies are a prevalent research topic today. Treatments such as stem cell therapy and platelet-rich plasma are among the vascular-regenerative treatments. Regenerative therapies are tried in urology practice, especially in erectile dysfunction, where vascular pathology is common. At the same time, it is used for urethral stricture disease, in which damaged urethral tissue heal with fibrosis.

After augmentation urethroplasty, spongiofibrosis may occur again, and treatment results may be adversely affected. Therefore, clinicians aim to improve urethral stricture treatment results with angiogenic therapies or tissue implants. Especially in recent years, bioengineered graft materials have been produced in tissue cultures. Using autologous bioengineered materials in treatments may be more advantageous than synthetic materials for foreign body reactions. In addition, bioengineering technology products can be edited, and they can improve

* Corresponding Author's Email: dr.emre5567@gmail.com.
† Corresponding Author's Email: yavuzilki@gmail.com.

In: Vascularization and Its Role in Medicine and Tissue Engineering
Editors: Emre Bulbul and Murat Oguz Ozilhan
ISBN: 979-8-89113-041-8

the efficacy and safety of treatments. Tissue-engineering techniques can also be used in penile length augmentation treatment.

Regenerative therapies can solve vascular problems in erectile dysfunction thanks to their neovascularization effects. Both regenerative therapy and tissue engineering can be applied as a component of minimally invasive treatments in treating urethral strictures. In addition, some studies continue to reduce the contraction of bioengineered graft materials in cell cultures.

Keywords: tissue engineering, endothelial dysfunction, bioengineered grafts, erectile dysfunction, regenerative therapies, penile enlargement

Introduction

Regenerative therapies and tissue engineering are used in many fields of medicine. Regenerative therapies are a prevalent research topic today. These treatments it is aimed to increase tissue healing by increasing vascularization. Regenerative therapies can solve vascular problems in erectile dysfunction thanks to their neovascularization effects. Both regenerative therapy and tissue engineering can be applied as a component of minimally invasive treatments in treating urethral strictures [1, 2]. The primary mechanism of these treatments is the stimulation of many growth factors and the occurrence of neovascularization. Treatments such as stem cell therapy (SCT) and platelet-rich plasma (PRP) are among the vascular-regenerative treatments.

Reconstructive implantations in urology are applied in a limited population, such as urethral stricture disease. Urethral stricture disease occurs due to spongiofibrosis. After augmentation urethroplasty, spongiofibrosis may occur again, and treatment results may be adversely affected. For this reason, there are no strong recommendations in the guidelines about the type of graft materials to be used in augmentation urethroplasty. Therefore, it is aimed to improve the treatment results of urethral stricture with alternative angiogenic therapies and tissue implants.

Especially in recent years, bioengineered graft materials have been produced in tissue cultures. However, there needs to be more data for evidence-based medicine applications due to the low number of patients in all these studies. At the same time, there needs to be more data on long-term results and safety, although it has been reported to be safe in some studies.

Neovascularization and Angiogenic Therapies in the Treatment of Erectile Dysfunction

Low-Intensity Extracorporeal Shock Wave Therapy and Neovascularization

Erectile dysfunction (ED) is subdivided into vascular and psychogenic. Phosphodiesterase type 5 inhibitors (PDE5i) are the primary treatment option for ED. The most noticeable effect of PDE5i is to provide vasodilation by increasing the amount of nitric oxide in the cavernosal vascular smooth muscle. With the relaxation in the corpus cavernosum, an erection occurs, and its continuity is ensured. In addition, low-intensity extracorporeal shock wave therapy (Li-ESWT) therapy has been reported to stimulate neovascularization and neuro-regeneration in ED patients [3, 4]. Therefore, Li-ESWT is recommended for the treatment of vasculogenic ED in the European Association of Urology guidelines [5].

Phosphodiesterase type 5 inhibitors and Li-ESWT can be used together due to synergistic effects. Karakose et al. compared patients who received only PDE5i and Li-ESWT plus PDE5i after radical prostatectomy. It was reported that patients receiving Li-ESWT plus PDE5i treatment had higher IIEF-5 scores at 6 and 12 months compared to those receiving PDE5i alone [6]. At the same time, it is stated that the neovascularization mechanism hypothesized in Li-ESWT treatment increases tissue regeneration [7]. In light of this hypothesis, it was stated that incontinence rates in patients who received Li-ESWT plus PDE5i treatment at six months were lower than those who received PDE5i treatment alone [6]. In addition, Li-ESWT is stated to be beneficial in chronic pelvic pain syndrome thanks to its positive vascular effects.

Mesenchymal Stem Cell and Platelet-Rich Plasma

There are many studies on the effectiveness of mesenchymal stem cell (MSC) and platelet-rich plasma (PRP) intracavernosal injection therapy in ED [8, 9]. MSC therapy methods include various derivations, such as human adipose tissue, bone marrow, and umbilical cord. MSC grafts can be obtained autologously or allograft. PRP can be easily obtained autologously from the patient's plasma. However, MSC production is more complex than PRP.

There is a hypothesis that mesenchymal stem cell therapy may be effective in neuronal, cellular, and vascular regeneration of the penis. Therefore, Ning et al. investigated the differentiation properties of adipose tissue-derived mesenchymal stem cells (AT-MSC) in rats. This study reported that AT-MSC differentiates into adipocytes, vascular smooth muscle cells, and neuronal cells in cell cultures [10]. Based on the present findings, in vivo studies are underway.

In vivo studies evaluate the clinical effect of intracavernosal MSC injection therapy on ED. Haahr et al. evaluated the effect of intracavernous injection of autologous AT-MSC therapy on ED after radical prostatectomy. It was stated that autologous intracavernous injection of AT-MSC therapy in continent patients significantly increased the International Index of Erectile Function-5 (IIEF-5) score at 12 months. However, there was no significant difference in the IIEF-5 score after AT-MSC therapy for incontinent and preoperative ED patients [11]. Therefore, according to this study, erectile functions can be better treated by considering the continence status of the patients.

The effect of therapies of MSCs of different origins on ED is a matter of curiosity. Yiou et al. administered intracavernosal bone marrow-derived mesenchymal stem cell therapy to 12 patients after radical prostatectomy. In the sixth month of evaluation, a significant improvement was detected in the scoring of the erectile function domain. No side effects were detected in an average of 62 months of follow-up. In addition, improvement in erectile function domain scores continued after long-term follow-up [12]. Levy et al. administered intracavernosal placental matrix−derived mesenchymal stem cells (PM-MSC) injection therapy to eight ED patients. 2 ml of isotonic serum was added to 1 ml of PM-MSC, and 1.5 ml was injected into each corpus cavernosum penis. There was an increase in the peak systolic velocity and end diastolic velocity measured at the third and sixth months in penile doppler ultrasonography. After this treatment, three patients did not require additional treatment for vaginal penetration. Four patients required oral medication, and one needed intracavernosal injection therapy for vaginal penetration. Three patients had mild erythema at the injection site, which resolved within 48 hours, and none had major complications [13]. Although the efficacy of these treatments is not yet apparent, they appear to be safe in the short term.

The etiology of ED may also affect the effectiveness of MSC therapies. The presence of both microvascular pathology and neurological pathology in diabetic patients may adversely affect the success of the treatment. Bahk et al. administered intracavernosal umbilical cord-derived MSC therapy to seven diabetic ED patients. It has been reported that there is an increase in erection in these patients, but not sufficient for vaginal penetration [14].

Platelet-rich plasma contains many platelet-derived growth factors. The most important are vascular endothelial growth and platelet-derived angiogenesis factors. For this reason, the efficacy and safety of PRP therapy in many diseases are being investigated [15, 16]. Protogerou et al. applied intracavernosal PRP plus AT-MSC to one group of ED patients and only PRP therapy to the other group. To obtain AT-MSC, adipose tissue was extensively washed with phosphate buffer saline after lipoaspiration. With this procedure, adipose tissue was cleared of erythrocytes. It was then treated with collagenase (Sigma-Aldrich, Darmstadt, Germany) and centrifuged at 500 gravity (g) for 6 minutes. After discarding the supernatant, the obtained pellet was placed in cell cultures (Costar, Corning Life, Canton, MA, USA). Subsequently, after several processes, they were transformed into AT-MSCs using the adipogenic differentiation kit (Ca. No. A1007001, Gibco, Thermo Fischer, Waltham, MA, USA). Finally, AT-MSCs were checked with immunohistochemical staining. While preparing the PRP, 20 ccs of blood samples were obtained from the patients and centrifuged at 160 g for 20 minutes.

After the platelet layer was isolated, a second centrifugation was performed at 450 g. AT-MSC was suspended in 2 ml of PRP solution after centrifugation. Intracavernosal AT-MSC plus PRP was applied to one group, and only PRP therapy to the other group. At three months, the IIEF-5 scores increased significantly in both groups. However, the two groups had no significant difference regarding IIEF-5 scores. No complications were detected in the short term. According to this study, intracavernosal AT-MSC plus was not superior to PRP and PRP therapy alone [17]. Consequently, PRP therapy seems promising in treating ED as an efficacy.

Angiogenic Therapies and Bioengineering in Urethral Stricture

The urethral stricture occurs due to severe spongiofibrosis. The spongiofibrosis (in the corpus spongiosum) present in the nature of the disease can cause recurrent urethral strictures. In treating urethral stricture, urethral dilatation or internal urethrotomy operations under direct vision can be performed using minimally invasive methods. In minimally invasive surgeries, the success rate is low as recurrence is common. In these treatments, it has been reported that while the success rate is 60% in strictures smaller than 2 cm in long-term follow-up, it is approximately 25% in strictures larger than

2 cm [18]. Because in urethrotomy performed under direct vision, the transurethral incision also heals with spongiofibrosis.

Urethroplasty is recommended for strictures that recur in the early period after minimally invasive surgery in case of stricture longer than 2 cm, located distally, multiple, severe spongiofibrosis, and history of multiple internal urethrotomy. [19]. Anastomotic urethroplasty can be applied in a limited group of patients (small urethral strictures: 1-2 cm). Generally, augmentation urethroplasty is required by using grafts or flaps in urethroplasty. It has been reported that there is no difference in terms of success between using grafts or flaps in augmentation urethroplasty. The augmentation urethroplasty success rate is approximately 85% [20].

The graft is mainly used in augmentation urethroplasty because it causes fewer donor area complications. Graft materials are used, such as oral mucosa, bladder mucosa, lingual mucosa, labial mucosa, penile skin, and scrotum skin, in augmentation urethroplasty. However, buccal mucosa grafts are the most widely used graft material today because they do not contain hair, are easy to prepare, have fewer donor area complications, and have good tissue quality.

Grafts can undergo contraction due to their histomorphological structure. Although graft contraction is a physiological process, it can affect the operation's success. Due to these contractions, the graft area may decrease, and the urethral stricture may recur after augmentation urethroplasty. For this reason, the choice of graft material, sufficient tissue content, and graft quality have a significant place in the operation's success. Graft contraction is divided into primary and secondary. Primary contraction takes place after the first harvest from the donor area. Primary contraction occurs more in the dermis of skin grafts than other grafts since the elastin content is higher. As the thickness of the skin grafts decreases, the primary contraction decreases. Thin grafts containing only the epidermis do not undergo primary contraction [21]. After the grafts are implanted in the targeted part, secondary contraction occurs. Split-thickness skin grafts are higher in secondary contraction than full-thickness skin grafts [22]. Because of the dermal fibrosis and high elastin content of the skin grafts, mucosal grafts are more often used for augmentation urethroplasty.

Patient and graft-related factors affect the contraction of the graft in urethroplasty operations. Graft contraction is affected by patient-related variables such as stricture length, localization, etiology, the blood supply to the graft bed, systemic diseases, and patient age. Graft-related factors are the type of graft and the quality of the graft (may depend on the surgeon who obtained the graft and the quality of the tissue from which the graft was taken).

Regenerative Therapies

Regenerative therapies are applied to the submucosal area perioperatively to reduce urethral stricture recurrence in patients who underwent internal urethrotomy under direct vision. Autologous PRP can be easily obtained from a blood sample with a centrifuge device. PRP contains abundant matrix proteins and growth factors that play a role in wound healing. Rezai et al. performed internal urethrotomy under direct vision in 87 patients with bulbar urethral strictures (smaller than 1.5 cm). They randomized these patients into two groups and applied submucosal autologous PRP to one group and normal saline (control group) to the other group in the same session. In patients who received submucosal autologous PRP or normal saline injection, urethral stricture recurrence rates at 24 months were 21% and 43%, respectively. When the lengths of urethral stricture recurrences were evaluated, the mean lengths of urethral stricture were 6.6 mm and 9.2 mm in PRP and control group patients, respectively. The mean calibration of strictures in PRP and control group patients were 9.5 Fr and 6.4 Fr, respectively. There was no significant difference between the two groups regarding complication rates [23]. In the literature, submucosal PRP's long-term efficacy and safety in treating urethral strictures are not apparent. However, since it is an autologous material, it seems safer than other synthetic derivative materials. Therefore, it is a great advantage that it can be applied as a component of minimally invasive surgery.

Mesenchymal Stem Cells

Some types of MSC are being investigated in the treatment of urethral strictures. Castiglione et al. investigated the effect of AT-MSC on urethral stricture in a rat model. A rat urethral stricture model was created with human recombinant transforming growth factor-b1 (TGF-β1) (PeproTech, NJ, USA) injected into the urethral wall. Subcutaneous adipose tissue was collected by lipoaspiration, and AT-MSC was characterized by flow cytometry. It was observed that the typical structure of the corpus spongiosum urethra was preserved in rats injected with AT-MSC into the urethral wall. At the same time, it was determined that inducible nitric oxide synthases and endothelial nitric oxide synthase expression increased in the rat urethral wall with submucosal AT-MSC therapy. In addition, it was found that the amount of collagen III and collagen I decreased in the rat urethral wall with submucosal AT-MSC therapy [24]. Increasing NO concentration and decreasing the amount of collagen can reduce spongiofibrosis. In conclusion, submucosal AT-MSC injection may reduce urethral stricture recurrence.

It is stated that genetic changes can occur at the cell level with MSC therapy. Liang et al. investigated the effect of umbilical cord-derived mesenchymal stem cells (UC-MSC) therapy in rats with urethral strictures. Rats with TGF-β1-induced urethral stricture were divided into groups of rats with UC-MSC therapy cultured with tumor necrosis factor-alpha (TNF-α) and rats with urethral stricture with only UC-MSC therapy. It was observed that urethral fibrosis was less in rats with UC-MSC therapy cultured with TNF-α to the urethral wall compared to those with only UC-MSC therapy. At the same time, miR-146a (an anti-inflammatory miRNA) was found to be selectively packaged in exosomes and expressed at a higher rate in rats with UC-MSC therapy cultured with TNF-α. It was stated that exosomes containing miR-146a suppressed the inflammatory response by inhibiting fibroblast activation. In conclusion, urethral fibrosis was reduced with a series of genetic changes in rats with UC-MSC therapy cultured with TNF-α [25]. According to this study, it may be possible to reduce recurrent spongiofibrosis by submucosal UC-MSC therapy cultured with TNF-α.

Bioengineered Grafts

Spongiofibrosis developing in urethral strictures can be reduced with MSC therapy. Liu et al. treated rats with urethral strictures using bone marrow-derived mesenchymal stem cells in augmentation urethroplasty. Bioengineered grafts were formed by seeding bone marrow-derived mesenchymal stem cells into synthetic cultures. After examining the augmented tissues, they reported a decrease in cytokines predisposing to fibrosis, such as IL-1β and TNF-α [26]. Bioengineered grafts cultured with MSC showed their effect by reducing spongiofibrosis in rats with urethral stricture. However, there are no adequate clinical studies of bioengineered grafts cultured with MSC. Therefore, the efficacy and safety of MSCs on humans are still curious.

Contraction at the cellular level occurs due to the contraction of actin filaments after the transformation of fibroblasts into myofibroblasts. Granulation tissue in the wound bed also can contract due to myofibroblasts. Keratinocyte cells have strong contractile adhesion connections and collagen fibers. Harrison et al. developed a model of human dermis-derived skin using 3D tissue engineering. In this model, keratinocytes and fibroblasts are seeded by increasing the number of cells with a series of processes. It is then placed in cell cultures. When β-aminopropionitrile (lysyl oxidase inhibitor) is used in cultures, it is seen that contraction decreases. It is stated that insulin-like growth factor-1, fibroblast growth factor, TNF-α, and prostaglandin-E2 do not affect contraction in cultures. A significant increase in contraction is seen when estriol is used in cultures [27]. Contraction of the tissue-engineered skin can be reduced by suturing it to a rigid frame for a few days [28].

Tissue engineering applications are becoming popular in modern medicine. For the first time, Bhargava et al. used tissue engineering to treat urethral strictures. In five patients, the augmentation urethroplasty was performed with bioengineered scaffold grafts originating from buccal mucosa. It was reported that urethral stricture recurrence occurred in two patients after urethroplasty [29]. The other three patients had no fibrosis or contraction during their 9-year follow-up [30].

The success of minimally invasive treatment of urethral stricture is low. Scott et al. bioengineered liquid buccal mucosa graft injection was applied to rabbits simultaneously with internal urethrotomy under direct vision. Rabbits who received a bioengineered liquid buccal mucosa graft injection (into the internal urethrotomy incision area) had a 58% recovery compared to 38% in those who underwent internal urethrotomy under direct vision only [31].

There are studies to improve minimally invasive treatment outcomes. Vaddi et al. used liquid bioengineered grafts originating from the buccal mucosa in the minimally invasive treatment of urethral stricture. They took an autologous buccal mucosal biopsy from patients and isolated epithelial cells. Isolated epithelial cells were cultured in a laboratory medium. Patients with urethral stricture underwent internal urethrotomy, and bioengineered liquid buccal mucosa grafts were perioperatively injected into the submucosal urethra. In this study, a copolymer with heat sensitive polymer component (poly [N-isopropyl acrylamide-co-n-butyl methacrylate] poly [NIPAAm-co-BMA]) and hydrophilic polymer component (polyethylene glycol) was used. Bioengineered polymers were formed by seeding buccal mucosal epithelial samples into these heat-regulated polymers. Six patients had penobulbar stenosis 2-3.5 cm in diameter, and internal urethrotomy was performed under direct vision. Simultaneously, urethroscopy was performed with a 17 Fr urethra-cystoscopy, and bioengineered gelation polymer was applied to the entire urethrotomy area with a 5 Fr ureteral catheter. Bioengineered polymers, in liquid form outside the body, transformed into solid form after submucosal injection and formed a fixed tissue. Two patients (33%) (one at 18 months and the other at 24 months) had a recurrence of urethral strictures at a 3-year follow-up [32]. Because submucosal injection of bioengineered liquid grafts is minimally invasive, this technique may be an excellent alternative to augmentation urethroplasty.

Experience in the use of bioengineered graft materials is increasing. Ram-Liebig et al. published the most extensive tissue engineering study in treating urethral strictures. In this study involving 99 patients from eight centers, an industrial product, autologous buccal mucosa-derived bioengineered scaffold graft (MukoCell®, UroTiss GmbH, Germany) was implanted in augmentation urethroplasty. With a certification system established in Germany, an authorized urologist received the buccal mucosa graft. Later, the buccal mucosa graft was sent to the firm. Bioengineered scaffold production by the company was used in augmentation urethroplasty within 48 hours after packaging. The success rate of augmentation urethroplasty with bioengineered graft scaffolds at 24 months was 62% [33].

Efficiency can be increased in augmentation urethroplasty with bioengineered grafts with different tissue origins. Raya-Rivera et al. used bioengineered grafts from bladder urothelium in augmentation urethroplasty. A biopsy was taken from the bladder, and urothelial tissue was obtained. Afterwards, epithelial and muscle cells were separated by a series of procedures. Epithelial cells were seeded on the inner-luminal surface of the tubular mesh with biodegradable polyglycolic acid (PGA; Sherwood Medical, St Louis, MO, USA). Muscle cells were planted on their outer surface, and scaffolds were formed. Bioengineered scaffold grafts were implanted in five patients in augmentation urethroplasty. Recurrence of urethral stricture was observed in only one patient, and an internal urethrotomy was performed under direct vision in the fourth week. The urethral biopsies taken in the third month determined that the grafts showed a typical urothelium structure. No other patients had a recurrence of urethral strictures at approximately six years of follow-up [28]. Fossum et al. used bioengineered grafts from bladder urothelium in pediatric augmentation urethroplasty. First, urothelial cells were obtained by bladder washing. Then, three weeks before the operation, the acellular dermis was prepared in the tissue engineering laboratory by removing epithelium and antigen. Urothelium cells were lysed and seeded on acellular dermis culture. Autologous bioengineered grafts were prepared by preserving the collagen structure. Augmentation urethroplasty was performed in six pediatric patients using a bioengineered graft. At a mean follow-up of seven years, only one patient had a urethral stricture recurrence and underwent direct vision internal urethrotomy at 12 months [34]. Bioengineered grafts originating from the bladder urothelium can be better adapted with their structural similarity to the urethra.

Adjustments can reduce the contraction of bioengineered graphs in cell culture. Patterson et al. reported that in bioengineered tissue cultures originating from the buccal mucosa, 45% surface reduction was observed in the fourth week due to contraction. Adding glutaraldehyde to bioengineered tissue cultures showed a significant reduction in cell contraction. Thanks to glutaraldehyde, only 5% of the surface area was lost. Surface area loss in tissue culture bioengineered with mechanical restraint and β-aminopropionitrile was 21% and 28%, respectively. These techniques for reducing contraction did not show any loss of viability of bioengineered tissue culture cells [35].

Bioengineered grafts are being investigated for less contraction. Simsek et al. compared bioengineered scaffold grafts originating from the natural dermis and buccal mucosa. They obtained biopsies of buccal mucosa from volunteers. After a series of procedures, keratinocytes were obtained from the lower part of the epidermis and the upper part of the dermis with the help of a scalpel. Fibroblasts were obtained from the remaining dermal tissue. After a series of procedures, fibrous mats were collected from Poly-L-lactic acid (PLA) and Poly-3-hydroxybutyrate-co-3-Hydroxyvalerate (PHBV) (Goodfellow, Cambridge, U.K.) scaffolds and monolayer scaffolds were formed. After a series of processes, trilayer scaffolds were formed using micro-fibrous PLA and nano-fibrous PHBV scaffolds. Trilayer (PLA-PHBV-PLA) and monolayer (PLA, PHBV) electrospun scaffolds were seeded with 150,000 fibroblasts and then 300,000 keratinocytes. In addition, 150,000 fibroblasts and then 300,000 keratinocytes were seeded into the Euro skin dermis. As a result, it was determined that the ultimate tensile strength of PLA scaffolds was lower than Euro skin. The ultimate tensile strength of trilayer scaffolds was lower than other scaffolds. Trilayer micro-nano-3D scaffolds were found to have a minimum contraction rate. Trilayer micro-nano-3D scaffolds were favourable for cell viability, keratinocyte, and fibroblast growth [36]. Trilayer scaffolds may stimulate the immunological system less in urethral reconstruction, as they will have fewer antigens than the oral mucosa. This way, the applied graft reconstruction can detect a better immunological adaptation to the tissue and the body.

Bioengineered graft materials show promise for augmentation urethroplasty. Although tissue engineering produces graft material for augmentation urethroplasties, it does not yet significantly reduce urethral stricture recurrence. However, in vitro studies continue to reduce the contraction of tissue-engineered graft materials. Today, the use of tissue-engineered graft materials remains to be determined regarding long-term success and complications. Therefore, tissue-engineered graft materials can be used with caution in urethral augmentation.

Vascular Regenerative Therapies and Tissue Engineering for Penile Augmentation

Who Has Penile Enlargement Surgery?

There is no consensus on the definition of the small penis [37]. In measurements, the fat pad should be retracted towards the pubic bone at the junction of the pubic bone and penile skin. Flaccid penile length is the measurement of the dorsal skin of the penis from the junction of the pubic bone and penile skin to the meatus. Stretched penile length is the measurement of the dorsal skin of the penis from the junction of the pubic bone and penile skin to the meatus by gentle manual stretching of the glans penis. It is stated that stretched penile length and erect penile length are correlated with each other. However, the relationship between flaccid penile length and erect penile length is unclear [38, 39]. The true micropenis is considered to be <4 cm flaccid and <7.5 cm when stretched or erect [40]. Some patients think their penis is small despite having a standard penis size. This condition is defined as small penis anxiety [41]. Body dysmorphic disorder (BDD) is defined as experiencing at least one hour a day, continuing obsessive behaviours in follow-up examinations, and causing significant psychological distress [42]. Before these patients are evaluated for penile length augmentation treatment, because of the risk of suicide, they should be referred for psychological evaluation and counselling. Penile length augmentation treatments are generally applied to both true micropenis and BDD patients with standard penis sizes.

Which Tissue or Synthetic Materials Are Used for Penile Augmentation Surgery?

Autologous grafts, biological, synthetic filling materials injection, and synthetic implants are used in penile augmentation surgery. Autologous implantation of cartilage graft to tunica albuginea, acellular dermal matrix, free dermal-fat graft, and free fat penile subcutaneous injections are used. As biological material, the implantation of bioengineered biodegradable scaffolds to tunica albuginea and penile subcutaneous injections of hyaluronic acid and collagen can be applied. These autologous and biological materials can be resorbed in less than one year. Calcium hydroxyapatite, poly-lactic acid, and dextran from synthetic filling materials can be resorbed in about two years. Permanent synthetic filling materials are polymethylmethacrylate microspheres, polyacrylamide hydrogel, and silicone [43]. A penile-length silicone implant can also be applied in penile augmentation by implanting in the tunica albuginea [44].

How Long Does Penis Enlargement Surgery Lengthen the Penis?

Penile augmentation surgery provides mainly flaccid penile length and girth increase. Although developments in surgical methods continue, the increase in erect penile girth and length is minimal in many techniques. Penile-length silicone implants, bioengineered biodegradable scaffold implantation, autologous cartilage implantation, and free dermal-fat graft strip methods are reported as the most valuable methods. While there is a gain of approximately 2 cm in flaccid penis length with ligamentolysis, there is no significant gain in erected penile length [39]. Penile subcutaneous filler injection increases penile girth but does not increase penile length. In light of this information, preoperative awareness and postoperative satisfaction can be increased by providing detailed information to patients in penile augmentation surgeries.

When the autologous cartilage graft is implanted into the corpus cavernosum, an actual length of approximately 3 cm in flaccid and erect penis length is increased. In addition, the penile subcutaneous tissue flap is turned around the autologous cartilage graft, creating a vascular bed. Postoperative follow-up imaging shows that this vascular bed preserves the viability of the graft [45].

Penile-length silicone implant surgery, implanted in the tunica albuginea with a mesh, has recently been used and provides significant gains. Ellist et al. reported that penile-length silicone implant surgery has successful and safe long-term results. [46]. Flaccid penile girth and penile length increase with the penile length of silicone implant was 4.9 cm and 2.2 cm, respectively.

Autologous adipose tissue obtained from the periumbilical and suprapubic regions is used as a graft. After free autologous fat grafting with V-Y plasty and suspensory ligament release, the increase in flaccid and erect penile length was 2.5 cm and 1 cm, respectively (at 12-month follow-up) [47]. It has been reported that the increase in erect penile length reaches up to 1.9 cm when the free dermal-fat graft strip method is combined with V-Y plasty and suspensory ligament release [48]. In addition, it has been reported that suprapubic panniculectomy contributes to the flaccid length of the penis [49].

Autologous free dermal graft obtained from the inguinal area is used in penile length augmentation surgery. The 0.2-0.4 cm thick dermal graft is implanted on the dorsal surface of the tunica albuginea from the proximal border of the penis to the sulcus coronarius, with the dermal surface up. The increase in flaccid and erect penile length with this method was 2 cm and 0.8 cm, respectively [50].

Injection of the penile subcutaneous biological or synthetic fillers increases penile girth. It is stated that there is no statistically significant difference between hyaluronic acid and polylactic acid fillers in terms of penile girth increase. However, in terms of flaccid penile girth increase, hyaluronic acid fillers (2.1 cm) provides a minimal advantage over polylactic acid (1.6 cm) fillers (at six months follow-up). Yang et al. reported that penile subcutaneous injection of cross-linked dextran and polymethylmethacrylate mixture provided a 3.8 cm flaccid penile girth increase (at six months) [51].

The Place of Tissue Engineering in Penile Augmentation Surgery

Bioengineered biodegradable scaffolds grafts can be used in penile augmentation surgery. First, the erythrocytes of the dermis tissue taken from the penis are removed. Then, it is incubated with collagenase type 4 and 5% CO2. The separated fibroblasts are suspended in a culture medium with 5% patient serum, and the number of cells increases. In about a month, fibroblast cells can be increased by up to 20 million. Next, polylactic-co-glycolic acid scaffold (PLGA, Regen Biotech Inc., Sungnam, Korea) is pretreated. In addition, the scaffold is incubated with 20 million fibroblasts. Finally, two seeded scaffolds are implanted between the dartos and buck fascias. It has been reported that penile sensitivity was not affected in this method, which provides penile girth enhancement in particular. At a mean follow-up of two years, 97% of patients reported satisfaction with the operation. In this method, flaccid and erected penile girth increases, 3.1 cm and 2.5 cm were obtained, respectively. In these patients who also underwent ligamentolysis, an increase of 3.5 cm and 0.7 cm in flaccid and erect penile length were achieved, respectively [52].

Is Penile Augmentation Surgery Safe?

The penile subcutaneous injection of the acellular dermal matrix has high complication rates in penile augmentation surgery. Penile subcutaneous injections of these fillers have complications such as surgical wound infection, purulent discharge, severe penile edema, and ulcerated penile skin lesions [53].

The results are controversial in the penile subcutaneous injection of liquid injectable silicone. While it is reported to be successful and safe in the short term [54], migratory and granulomatous complications may occur in the long term [55, 56].

Penile subcutaneous mineral oil (vaseline) and cod liver oil injections are made by non-medical persons or as self-injection. These injections can cause paraffinoma (granuloma). For this reason, they are not recommended [57, 58].

Conclusion

Regenerative therapies can solve vascular problems in erectile dysfunction thanks to their neovascularization effects. Using autologous bioengineered materials in treatments may be more advantageous than synthetic materials in foreign body reactions. In addition, bioengineering technology products can be edited, and they can improve the efficacy and safety of treatments. Both regenerative therapy and tissue engineering can be applied as a component of minimally invasive treatments in treating urethral strictures. Tissue-engineering techniques can also be used in penile length augmentation surgery. However, prospective studies in larger patient groups are needed for the efficacy and safety of regenerative therapies and tissue-engineering methods.

References

[1] Matz, E. L., Terlecki, R., Zhang, Y., Jackson, J., Atala, A. (2019). Stem cell therapy for erectile dysfunction. *Sexual medicine reviews*, *7*(2), 321-328.

[2] Aydın, A., Sönmez, M. G., Oltulu, P., Kocabaş, R., Sönmez, L. Ö., Özcan, S., Balasar, M. (2020). Histopathologic evaluation of the effects of intraurethral platelet-rich plasma in urethral trauma experimentally induced in rat model. *Urology*, *141*, 187-e9.

[3] Ito, K., Fukumoto, Y., Shimokawa, H. (2011). Extracorporeal shock wave therapy for ischemic cardiovascular disorders. *American Journal of Cardiovascular Drugs*, *11*(5), 295-302.

[4] Mense S, Hoheisel U. Shock wave treatment improves nerve regeneration in the rat. *Muscle Nerve*. 2013;47:702–10.

[5] Salonia A, Minhas S, Bettocchi C, Carvalho J, Corona G, Jones TH, Kadioglu A, Martinez-Salamanca JI, Serefoglu EC, Verze P. EAU guidelines on sexual and reproductive health. European association of urology guidelines. Edn. presented at *the EAU Annual Congress Milan* 2023. ISBN 978-94-92671-19-6.

[6] Karakose, A., Yitgin, Y. (2021). Penile rehabilitation with low-intensity extracorporeal shock wave therapy in patients after prostate cancer surgery. Early physiological changes and postoperative follow-up outcomes. *International Journal of Clinical Practice*, *75*(12), e14804.

[7] Hayashi D, Kawakami K, Ito K, Ishii K, Tanno H, Imai Y, Kanno E, Maruyama R, Shimokawa H, Tachi M. Low-energy extracorporeal shock wave therapy enhances skin wound healing in diabetic mice: A critical role of endothelial nitric oxide synthase. *Wound repair and regeneration*. 2012 Nov;20(6):887-895.

[8] Lin, C. S., Xin, Z. C., Wang, Z., Deng, C., Huang, Y. C., Lin, G., Lue, T. F. (2012). Stem cell therapy for erectile dysfunction: a critical review. *Stem cells and development*, *21*(3), 343-351.

[9] Epifanova, M. V., Gvasalia, B. R., Durashov, M. A., Artemenko, S. A. (2020). Platelet-rich plasma therapy for male sexual dysfunction: myth or reality? *Sexual Medicine Reviews*, *8*(1), 106-113.

[10] Ning H, Lin G, Lue TF, Lin CS. Neuron-like differentiation of adipose tissue derived stromal cells and vascular smooth muscle cells. *Differentiation*. 2006;74:510–8.

[11] Haahr MK, Jensen CH, Toyserkani NM, Andersen DC, Damkier P, Sørensen JA, Sheikh SP, Lund L. A 12-month follow-up after a single intracavernous injection of autologous adipose-derived regenerative cells in patients with erectile dysfunction following radical prostatectomy: an open-label phase I clinical trial. *Urology*. 2018 Nov 1;121:203-e6.

[12] Yiou, R., Hamidou, L., Birebent, B., Bitari, D., Le Corvoisier, P., Contremoulins, I., Rouard, H. (2017). Intracavernous injections of bone marrow mononucleated cells for postradical prostatectomy erectile dysfunction: final results of the INSTIN clinical trial. *European urology focus*, *3*(6), 643-645.

[13] Levy JA, Marchand M, Iorio L, Cassini W, Zahalsky MP. Determining the feasibility of managing erectile dysfunction in humans with placental-derived stem cells. *J Osteopath Med*. 2016;116:e1–e5.

[14] Bahk JY, Jung JH, Han H, Min SK, Lee YS. Treatment of diabetic impotence with umbilical cord blood stem cell intracavernosal transplant: preliminary report of 7 cases. *Exp Clin Transpl*. 2010;8:150–60.

[15] Albanese, A., Licata, M. E., Polizzi, B., Campisi, G. (2013). Platelet-rich plasma (PRP) in dental and oral surgery: from the wound healing to bone regeneration. *Immunity & Ageing*, *10*(1), 1-10.

[16] Bos-Mikich, A., De Oliveira, R., Frantz, N. (2018). Platelet-rich plasma therapy and reproductive medicine. *Journal of assisted reproduction and genetics*, *35*(5), 753-756.

[17] Protogerou V, Michalopoulos E, Mallis P, Gontika I, Dimou Z, Liakouras C, Stavropoulos-Giokas C, Kostakopoulos N, Chrisofos M, Deliveliotis C. Administration of adipose derived mesenchymal stem cells and platelet lysate in erectile dysfunction: a single center pilot study. *Bioengineering*. 2019 Mar 5;6(1):21.

[18] Steenkamp JW, Heyns CF, De Kock ML. Internal urethrotomy versus dilation as treatment for male urethral strictures: a prospective, randomized comparison. *J Urol* 1997;157:98e101.

[19] Simsek, A., Aldamanhori, R., Chapple, C. R., MacNeil, S. (2018). Overcoming scarring in the urethra: Challenges for tissue engineering. *Asian Journal of Urology*, 5(2), 69-77.

[20] Wessells H, McAninch JW. Current controversies in anterior urethral stricture repair: free-graft versus pedicled skin-flap reconstruction. *World J Urol* 1998; 16:175e80.

[21] Davis JS, Kitlowski EA. The Immediate contraction of cutaneous grafts and its cause. *Arch Surg* 1931;23:954e65.

[22] Rudolph R. The effect of skin graft preparation on wound contraction. *Surg Gynecol Obstet* 1976;142:49e56.

[23] Rezaei M, Badiei R, Badiei R: The effect of platelet-rich plasma injection on post-internal urethrotomy stricture recurrence. *World J Urol*. 2019; 37(9): 1959–1964.

[24] Castiglione F, Dewulf K, Hakim L, Weyne E, Montorsi F, Russo A, Boeri L, Bivalacqua TJ, De Ridder D, Joniau S, Albersen M. Adipose-derived stem cells counteract urethral stricture formation in rats. *European urology*. 2016 Dec 1;70(6): 1032-1041.

[25] Liang YC, Wu YP, Li XD, Chen SH, Ye XJ, Xue XY, Xu N. TNF-α-induced exosomal miR-146a mediates mesenchymal stem cell-dependent suppression of urethral stricture. *Journal of Cellular Physiology*. 2019 Dec;234(12):23243-23255.

[26] Liu JS, Bury MI, Fuller NJ, Sturm RM, Ahmad N, Sharma AK. Bone marrow stem/progenitor cells attenuate the inflammatory milieu following substitution urethroplasty. *Scientific reports*. 2016 Oct 20;6(1):1-7.

[27] Harrison CA, Gossiel F, Layton CM, Bullock AJ, Johnson T, Blumsohn A, MacNeil S. Use of an in vitro model of tissue-engineered skin to investigate the mechanism of skin graft contraction. *Tissue engineering*. 2006 Nov 1;12(11):3119-3133.

[28] Raya-Rivera A, Esquiliano DR, Yoo JJ, Lopez-Bayghen E, Soker S, Atala A. Tissue-engineered autologous urethras for patients who need reconstruction: an observational study. *Lancet* 2011;377:1175e82.

[29] Bhargava S, Patterson JM, Inman RD, MacNeil S, Chapple CR. Tissue-engineered buccal mucosa urethroplasty-clinical outcomes. *Eur Urol* 2008;53:1263e9.

[30] Osman NI, Patterson JM, MacNeil S, Chapple CR. Long-term follow-up after tissue-engineered buccal mucosa urethroplasty. *Eur Urol* 2014;66:790e1.

[31] Scott KA, Li G, Manwaring J, Nikolavsky DA, Fudym Y, Caza T, Badar Z, Taylor N, Bratslavsky G, Kotula L, Nikolavsky D. Liquid buccal mucosa graft endoscopic

urethroplasty: a validation animal study. *World Journal of Urology*. 2020 Sep;38: 2139-2145.

[32] Vaddi SP, Reddy VB, Abraham SJK: Buccal Epithelium Expanded and Encapsulated in Scaffold-Hybrid Approach to Urethral Stricture (BEES-HAUS) Procedure: A Novel Cell Therapy-Based Pilot Study. *Int J Urol*. 2019; 26(2): 253–257.

[33] Ram-Liebig G, Barbagli G, Heidenreich A, Fahlenkamp D, Romano G, Rebmann U, Standhaft D, Van Ahlen H, Schakaki S, Balsmeyer U, Spiegler M. Results of use of tissue-engineered autologous oral mucosa graft for urethral reconstruction: a multicenter, prospective, observational trial. *EBioMedicine*. 2017 Sep 1;23:185-192.

[34] Fossum, M., Skikuniene, J., Orrego, A., Nordenskjöld, A. (2012). Prepubertal follow-up after hypospadias repair with autologous in vitro cultured urothelial cells. *Acta paediatrica*, 101(7), 755-760.

[35] Patterson JM, Bullock AJ, MacNeil S, Chapple CR. Methods to reduce the contraction of tissue-engineered buccal mucosa for Use in substitution urethroplasty. *Eur Urol* 2011;60:856e61.

[36] Simsek, A., Bullock, A. J., Roman, S., Chapple, C. R., Macneil, S. (2018). Developing improved tissue-engineered buccal mucosa grafts for urethral reconstruction. *Canadian Urological Association Journal*, *12*(5), E234.

[37] Ghanem H, Glina S, Assalian P, Buvat J. Position paper: management of men complaining of a small penis despite an actually normal size. *J Sex Med*. 2013;10:294–303.

[38] Davoudzadeh EP, Davoudzadeh NP, Margolin E, Stahl PJ, Stember DS. Penile length: measurement technique and applications. *Sex Med Rev*. 2018;6:261–271.

[39] García Gómez, B., Alonso Isa, M., García Rojo, E., Fiorillo, A., Romero Otero, J. (2022). Penile length augmentation surgical and non-surgical approaches for aesthetical purposes. *International Journal of Impotence Research*, *34*(4), 332-336.

[40] Wessells H, Lue TF, McAninch JW. Penile length in the flaccid and erect states: guidelines for penile augmentation. *J Urol*. 1996;156:995–997.

[41] Wylie KR, Eardley I. Penile size and the "small penis syndrome." *BJU Int*. 2007;99:1449–1455.

[42] Marra G, Drury A, Tran L, Veale D, Muir GH. Systematic review of surgical and nonsurgical interventions in normal men complaining of small penis size. *Sex Med Rev*. 2020;8:158–180.

[43] Abo-Hedibah, S. A., Badawi, A. N., Aly, S. A., Ismail, S. R., Elmokadem, A. H. (2021). Penile girth augmentation by injectable fillers: a comprehensive review of imaging features and inflammatory complications. *Abdominal Radiology*, *46*(4), 1703-1717.

[44] Wilson, S. K., Picazo, A. L. L. (2022). Update on the Penuma® an FDA-cleared penile implant for aesthetic enhancement of the flaccid penis. *International Journal of Impotence Research*, 34(4), 369-374.

[45] Perovic, S. V., Djordjevic, M. L. J. (2000). Penile lengthening. *BJU international*, *86*(9), 1028-1033.

[46] Elist, J. J., Valenzuela, R., Hillelsohn, J., Feng, T., Hosseini, A. (2018). A single-surgeon retrospective and preliminary evaluation of the safety and effectiveness of

the penuma silicone sleeve implant for elective cosmetic correction of the flaccid penis. *The Journal of Sexual Medicine*, 15(9), 1216-1223.

[47] Littara, A., Melone, R., Morales-Medina, J. C., Iannitti, T., Palmieri, B. (2019). Cosmetic penile enhancement surgery: a 3-year single-centre retrospective clinical evaluation of 355 cases. *Scientific Reports*, 9(1), 1-10.

[48] Xu, L., Zhao, M., Yang, Z., Chen, W., Li, Y., Ma, N., Ma, T. (2016). Modified penile augmentation by dermal-fat graft in post-hypospadias adults. *Aesthetic plastic surgery*, 40(1), 120-129.

[49] Zhang, X., Huang, Z., Xiao, Y., Kuang, L., Zhang, M., Zhang, G., Xu, T. (2019). Suspensory ligament release combined with acellular dermal matrix filler in infrapubic space: a new method for penile length augmentation. *Andrologia*, 51(9), e13351.

[50] Zhang, G. X., Weng, M., Wang, M. D., Bai, W. J. (2016). Autologous dermal graft combined with a modified degloving procedure for penile augmentation in young adults: a preliminary study. *Andrology*, *4*(5), 927-931.

[51] Yang, D. Y., Lee, W. K., Kim, S. C. (2013). Tolerability and efficacy of newly developed penile injection of cross-linked dextran and polymethylmethacrylate mixture on penile enhancement: 6 months follow-up. *International Journal of Impotence Research*, 25(3), 99-103.

[52] Perovic, S. V., Byun, J. S., Scheplev, P., Djordjevic, M. L., Kim, J. H., Bubanj, T. (2006). New perspectives of penile enhancement surgery: tissue engineering with biodegradable scaffolds. *European urology*, *49*(1), 139-147.

[53] Tealab, A. A., Maarouf, A. M., Habous, M., Ralph, D. J., Abohashem, S. (2013). The Use of an acellular collagen matrix in penile augmentation: A pilot study in Saudi Arabia. *Arab Journal of Urology*, *11*(2), 169-173.

[54] Yacobi Y, Tsivian A, Grinberg R, Kessler O. Short-term results of incremental penile girth enhancement using liquid injectable silicone: Words of praise for a change. *Asian journal of andrology.* 2007 May;9(3):408-413.

[55] Silberstein J, Downs T, Goldstein I (2008) Penile injection with silicone: case report and review of the literature. *J Sex Med* 5:2231–2237.

[56] Shaeer, O., Shaeer, K. (2009). Delayed complications of gel injection for penile girth augmentation. *The Journal of Sexual Medicine*, *6*(7), 2072-2078.

[57] Akkus, E., Iscimen, A., Tasli, L., Hattat, H. (2006). Paraffinoma and ulcer of the external genitalia after self-injection of Vaseline. *The Journal of Sexual Medicine*, 3(1), 170-172.

[58] Al-Ansari, A. A., Shamsodini, A., Talib, R. A., Gul, T., Shokeir, A. A. (2010). Subcutaneous cod liver oil injection for penile augmentation: review of literature and report of eight cases. *Urology*, 75(5), 1181-1184.

Index

M

N

O

P

R

S

T

About the Editors

Emre Bulbul, MD

Department of Urology

Vakfikebir State Hospital/Trabzon, Turkey

Email: dr.emre5567@gmail.com.

Education: Cerrahpaşa Faculty of Medicine, Department of Urology 2014-2020.

Honors and awards: 5. Ürolojik Cerrahi Derneği Kongresi (Turkey Urological Surgery Congress), 2020, Third prize in Minimally Invasive Urology Presentations.

Publications from the Last 3 Years:

1. Onal, B., Abdullahoglu, D., Bulbul, E., Kırlı, E. A., Ilki, F. Y. (2020). Abdominal Wall Retraction Sutures for Laparoscopic Trocar Insertion in Children. *Videourology*, 34(6). https://doi.org/10.1089/vid.2020.0051.
2. Bulbul, E., Ilki, F. Y., Gultekin, M. H., Erozenci, A., Tutar, O., Citgez, S., Onal, B. (2021). Ureteral wall thickness is an independent parameter affecting the success of extracorporeal shock wave lithotripsy treatment in ureteral stones above the iliac crest. *International Journal of Clinical Practice*, e14264.
3. 3-Bulbul, E., Ilki, F. Y., Zengin, A. K., Ozden, S. B., Ozbek, E. (2021). Insertion of Trocar into the Cyst for Laparoscopic Management of Hydatid Kidney Disease. *Videourology*, 35(6).
4. Kırlı, E. A., Bulbul, E., Kaygısız, O., Yeni, S., Can, G., Tutar, O., Onal, B. (2021). Ureteral wall thickness at the stone site: A critical predictor of success and complications in children undergoing semi-rigid ureteroscopy. *Journal of Pediatric Urology*, 17(6), 796-e1.

5. Ozman, O., Citgez, S., Bulbul, E., Sahin, K. C., Ozkara, H. (2021). *Is There Any Relationship Between Varicocele and Reproductive Hormone Status in Non-obstructive Azoospermia?*
6. Bulbul, E., Gultekin, M. H., Citgez, S., Derekoylu, E., Demirbilek, M., Akkus, E., Ozkara, H. (2022). Penile fracture: Tertiary care center experience and long-term complications after immediate repair. *Andrology*, 10(3), 560-566.
7. Bulbul, E., Aydin E, Yilmaz E. Evaluation of endothelial dysfunction with cardio-ankle vascular index measurements in patients with erectile dysfunction. *Andrology*. 2022 Jul;10(5):926-930. doi: 10.1111/andr.13191. Epub 2022 May 1. PMID: 35466575.
8. Ilki, F. Y., Bulbul, E., Gultekin MH, Citgez S, Demirdag C, Ozden SB, Onal B. Comparison of laparoscopic and open ureterolysis for retroperitoneal fibrosis: Results from a tertiary referral center. *Journal of Endourology*, 36(11), 1425-1430. doi: 10.1089/end.2022.0135. PMID: 35521656.
9. Bulbul E, Gultekin MH, Ilki FY Citgez, S Tutar, O, Onal, B. (2022). The Association Between Ureteral Wall Thickness and Need for Additional Procedures after Primary Ureteroscopy in Patients with Ureteral Stones above the Iliac Crest. *Aktuelle Urologie*, 54(01), 37-43.
10. Demirdag, C., Bulbul, E., Gultekin, M. H., Simsekoglu, M. F., Ilki, F. Y., Kalender, G., Citgez, S. (2023). Comparison of split-cuff nipple and modified Lich-Gregoir ureteroneocystostomy in iatrogenic distal ureteral injuries: tertiary care center experience. *International Urology and Nephrology*, 55(3), 605-611.
11. Ilki, Y., Bulbul, E., Gultekin, M. H., Erozenci, A., Tutar, O., Citgez, S., Onal, B. (2023). In-vivo or in-vitro stone attenuation: what is more valuable for the prediction of renal stone composition in non-contrast-enhanced abdominal computed tomography? *Aktuelle Urologie,* 54(01), 30-36.
12. Bulbul, E., Ozilhan, M. O., Sezer, A., Yetisen, M., Ilki, F. Y. (2023). Possible Clinical Benefits of Cardio-Ankle Vascular Index Measurement in Urological Diseases. *Vascular Health and Risk Management*, 19, 127-132.

Murat Oguz Ozilhan, MD
T. C. Ministry of Health Ankara City Hospital
Ankara, Turkey
Email: murat_ozilhan@hotmail.com